TRAPPED

Living with Non-Fluent Aphasia

D1522161

Kevin Sweeney

ISBN: 9798866318209

Printed in the United States of America

Published by: Bookmarketeers.com

For Kelly, Ryan, Timmy, and Matty
Whom I Love More Than Words Can Say

"When a sieve is shaken, the husks appear,
so do one's faults when one speaks."

Sirach 27:4

Introduction

The goals of this book are two-fold. First, I would like to inspire others. You can do this; keep trying and never give up. Each year 795,000 people in America will have strokes, and those who survive need to be prepared to fight for every yard. It helps if you are blessed with a strong support network, like me, but I would fight by myself, and you should too.

Second, I would like to demonstrate my sense of humor and determination to my friends and family. I am really in here, same as I ever was, though you cannot hear me, and I really will get it all back, though it is likely to take years. Maybe I will be driving again for my 50th Birthday.

I suffered two strokes on August 26th, 2020, just a month after my 46th birthday. I was on the couch at home, which was rare, and watching the Yankees, which is what I still tend to do with my free time. It is funny what I remember. I remember having the strokes, the ride in the Ambulance, and the first Hospital which I was in the Emergency Room at INOVA-Cornwall (In Northern Virginia), where I got my shot of tPA (about three hours after I had my strokes). A tPA shot is given to people having strokes. It is short for tissue plasminogen activator. It restores blood flow to the brain. I have often wondered would I have been better off if I had gotten that shot earlier, but they wanted to be sure I was having a stroke. I think the shot can be dangerous for people not having a stroke, i.e., people with normal blood flow to the brain.

I do not remember any of the next three weeks when I was in two ICUs and got a costly helicopter ride in between, but, as we shall see, I had an eventful few weeks. At one point on the 26th or the early morning of the 27th, I pulled out my tubes and IVs and tried to leave the ICU at INOVA Loudoun. One of these tubes was draining the swelling in my brain. I have also often wondered whether I would be better off if that tube stayed in. It does not surprise me that I tried to leave the hospital. I had never had time for this and was exceptionally busy (Chapter 2) when it happened.

We never found the actual cause of my strokes, true for roughly 25% of all strokes. A doctor at Johns Hopkins University came the closest when he said my strokes were likely caused by a blood clot traveling from my heart, through a hole in my heart, to my brain. The hole is called a PFO, short for Patent Foramen Ovale. PFOs are about as common as being left-handed, and, for most people, not me, they cause no problem. PFOs occur after birth when the foramen ovale fails to close. The foramen ovale is a hole in the wall between the left and right atria of every human fetus. This hole allows blood to bypass the fetal lungs, which cannot work until exposed to air. When a newborn takes its first breath, the foramen ovale closes, and within a few months, it has entirely sealed in about 75 percent of us.

In late August 2020, I really was fighting for my life and almost died. I have spent all the time since September 2020 battling back, re-learning how to do everything. My favorite example of re-learning everything, one that I have used often, is brushing your teeth, something I can do. Think of all the steps involved in brushing your teeth. I had to learn these and all other things again. This book is a part of my therapy. I have been recently told (January 2022) that anything that gets me to think, like writing a book, is a good thing.

I named this book *TRAPPED* because I often know what to say; I just cannot say it. I find this very frustrating because I used to be quite eloquent. In fact, there was a picture of me kissing the Blarney Stone at my desk at work. I still have the picture. Kissing the Blarney Stone is supposed to give one the gift of eloquence; maybe I should kiss it again. One piece of advice I got was to use small words. Well, that is great, it is only big words that come to mind, and I feel like I am shortchanging my conversation partner if I use short words.

Also frustrating is my current need to do all things slowly. I do everything more slowly now; in fact, a goal for 2022 is to get faster in all things. This is quite difficult for me as I used to do everything fast and still remember the way it was with 100% accuracy. I feel 90% of getting faster will come from learning to do things better. Only 10% will come from my improvement.

Currently, I am beset by many maladies. Foremost among these is that my left hand (and to a lesser extent my left leg) does not work. My left arm tends to fly out uncontrollably. This makes it very difficult to do even simple tasks that require two hands. I still have difficulty with simple chores that require two hands – like buttoning jeans, putting on a band-aid, or cleaning my glasses. So, I must concentrate very hard to make my left hand do what I want it to do.

Second, a particular sore point is typing. I used to type 55ish words a minute with both hands, without looking. That plummeted to 10-12 wpm only using my right hand and looking. This is particularly problematic when writing a book. Typing this all out is a real labor of love. Take heart because my New Year's Resolution was to type with both hands, and I always keep my New Year's Resolutions by reducing them to practice – making them part of the routine. I am typing this book with two hands.

Third, I was always nearsighted and started wearing glasses to correct this when I was 19. I have been wearing glasses constantly since I was about 21. I guess I am a good candidate for laser surgery, but I could never justify the cost, and the notion of someone sticking lasers in my eyes seemed intrusive – less so now for all I have been through. Simply put, I cannot see anything without my glasses. My vision has definitely gotten worse since the strokes. In fact, my Occupational Therapist, Laura, was very concerned with my vision. I think she was right.

Fourth, it really inconveniences my family and me that I cannot currently drive. The story of how I lost my license, completely unintended, is a funny one. I was too aggressive with my occupational driving test, in March 2021, and they (a private company) told the Virginia DMV that I failed, and the Virginia DMV took my license. I cannot tell you how inconvenient this is. There are two salient pieces of data. First, I commuted almost 80 miles roundtrip to work daily. Second, my sons are old enough to have a busy extracurricular schedule but, mostly, too young to drive. Shuttling me to work was mostly Kelly; shuttling the boys to practices and games is all Kelly. To add insult to injury, I was often the coach of my sons' teams, which allowed me to set a workable schedule, something that has completely gone out the window since late August 2020.

Finally, as I mentioned above, I cannot talk. It is very frustrating that I often know what to say; I just cannot say it. I guess this is so common with my type of stroke that it has a name, non-fluent aphasia. This occurs when the person knows what they want to say but cannot communicate it to others. When it is severe, it can inhibit speech completely. It is a bit of a misnomer to say I cannot talk; I can. It just requires an immense amount of preparation. For example, I usually verbally relay the plan for the day to Kelly first thing in the morning. We have a lot of moving parts, so the plan is very important. Well, I prepare for hours while she, and the rest of our time zone, is asleep. I tend to go over the plan for the day in my head, imaging what I will say. This malady named this book.

I am blessed to have a strong support network; I am willing to fight on my own, but I will not have to. Figure 1 should help. Kelly is my wife and partner in all things. We were married on July 22nd, 2000. I would really be lost without her. Ryan, Timmy, and Matty are our sons. All three play a boatload of extracurricular sports and are Altar Severs at St. Francis de Sales Roman Catholic Parish in Purcellville, Virginia. Ryan, the oldest, is currently 17. Timmy, who is the most like me, is currently 16. Matty, the youngest, is currently 12, going on 19.

Ryan plays baseball year-round and is a left-handed pitcher and first baseman, and he looks like me. I prayed hard for a left-handed pitcher and got one. He wants to play baseball in college. Getting him ready to compete at that level has been my life's work since 2005. In fact, most of the teams I coached (Chapters 2 and 4) were because he was on them. Timmy's best sport is running, and we live in the right place for that. The Loudoun Valley High School Boy's Cross-Country team has recently won National Championships. He is a sub six minute miler, like I was at that age. Timmy is also a great point guard in basketball and on LVHS's Junior Varsity team. The Varsity Basketball team is quite good too. Timmy, this year, gave up baseball to run full time. It was the right decision, but it broke my heart as baseball is my first love.

Matty is in 7th grade and plays both baseball (Babe Ruth League and Travel) and basketball. He is the least athletic of the Sweeney boys, but there is evidence he is the most intelligent. This year we got a letter from his principal extolling his all As a virtue. In fact, all three boys make straight As, and I would expect no less. Also, importantly, all three boys, far from being freaked out by the situation (which they easily could have been), have taken care of me and learned four important life lessons along the way (Chapter 7). One more important thing about my family at the outset, we fight as a team, always have, and always will.

Pat is my brother, and Jamie is his wife. Cody and Cooper are their college-age children. Jamie is an Elementary School Principal, and Pat manages construction projects. Chris is Kelly's brother, and Liz is his wife. Connor and Hannah are their young (less than seven years old) children. Chris works for the US Postal Service; Liz runs programs for developmentally delayed adults. I love them all, and I pray for them every night.

I worked at the Office of The Director of National Intelligence from 2010 to 2022 and the Directorate of Strategic and Operational Planning (DSOP) at The National Counterterrorism Center (NCTC) since 2017. There will be plenty of time for me to talk about my professional life below (Chapter 2). What I will say at the outset is that my bosses at DSOP, Kulika Frazier and Damon Stevens, were very supportive of me; in fact, all of DSOP was. I still retain all of my connections from my job, and have included them in Figure 1.

Kelly is a Psychologist for Fairfax County Schools. While I know a lot less about her professional circumstances, I can say that her employer has been very understanding of our situation. Kelly is currently a part-time employee as she deals with my situation. This is problematic for us because the rules, being what they are, imply that part-time years, for her, do not count toward retirement, something we take very seriously. We are nothing if we are not planners (Conclusion). Kelly plans on going back to full-time for the 2022-2023 academic year.

My parents are deceased (Chapter 2), but Kelly's parents are relatively young and in good health. John and Sue have been very supportive of me, but particularly of Kelly (as this happened to her too). It is not possible to overstate their role. I think the regular conversations on the phone (John and Sue are snowbirds from Long Island, New York, who winter in Florida) have really helped Kelly, and they have had some great ideas.

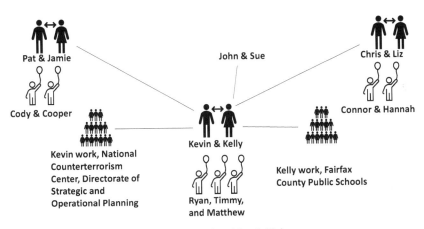

Figure 1 – My Work and Family Web

Figure 1: Family and Work Web

Plan of the book

Chapter 1 talks about my strokes as they happened. Chapter 2 details what I was at the time of my strokes. I was a lot and quite busy. There are some interesting stories there, and what I was in August 2020 was definitely, a product of where I came from. Chapter 3 talks about the weeks and months after August 26th. For the weeks thereafter, which I do not remember, I have had to rely on the recollections of my wife, Kelly. In Chapter 4, I will write about coaching Matty's Little League team in the Fall of 2021. I have reproduced for you all of my communications with the parents to demonstrate, hopefully, that I was having fun and wanted the kids to learn. I cannot tell you how many young men I have told to never give up. I guess what is good for the Goose is good for the Gander. Chapter 5 will talk about some of my more stellar accomplishments – which tend to cluster from November 2021 to February 2022; I started this book in January 2022. Chapter 6 talks about the now and what it is like to be me, I spend a lot of time talking about my typical day, and Chapter 7 is about four huge lessons my sons have learned from this experience, I also count my blessings there. I conclude with some general thoughts about going forward.

There are three categories of people I would like to thank. The first category is all those who helped me during my recovery. I am blessed, the list is long, and I have a lot of people to thank. I apologize if I forgot anyone, I tried to be comprehensive. I would like to thank Dr. Meagan Cooper at INOVA Cornwall, Dr. Cindy Lee ICU, Dr. Rana neurologist, and Cody ICU nurse at INOVA Loudoun. I am sorry I tried to leave the ICU. At INOVA Fairfax, where I spent some time, I would like to thank Dr. Choudhary neurology ICU, Dr. Ramesh ICU, Dr. Ashiny cardiologist, and nurses Evelyn, Kailyn, Angie, Molly, Courtney, and Crystal. I would also like to thank physician's assistants Karen, Jen, and Susan. At Encompass Health, where I did inpatient therapy, I would like to thank Maria Hurst, my case manager, Dr. Gaddipati, Aparma Iyer, for physical therapy, Michelle Villarreal, for speech therapy, and Nick Denizli for occupational therapy. Nick is noteworthy because I had my first showers with him, and he did not like my socks because they were hard to get on, which I kept, by the way. Spencer Neilson, James Marsh, Gerard Skinner, and

Kris Weshinsky visited me at home when I was at my Nadir; Kelly Gaffney, Gregg Burgess, Spencer Neilson, and Dale Weaver took me to lunch. These are all great people, but I would single out Dale; Dale Weaver is one of the best people around. The world would be a better place if there were more Dale Weavers in it. I should thank Erika, Krista, and Laurel, who gave me therapy at home. Krista recommended a bar for the bed, which I still use. For the longest time, a year, I have been an outpatient, and I should thank Dr. Shetal Patel, my general practitioner, Dr. Seth Tuwiner, my neurologist, whom I see about every two months and through whom I got to many of the doctors on this list, Dr. Nadim A. Geloo, a cardiologist who wanted to close the hole in my heart surgically and for whom I wore a heart monitor for 30 days in November and December of 2020, Dr. Mei Firestone, a hematologist, who looked in vain for a cause for my strokes in my blood ; Dr. Rafael Llinas, the neurologist at Johns Hopkins University who came the closest to nailing the cause of my strokes and the inspiration for this book; and my therapists who have helped me tremendously and whose many suggestions are all over this book Elisabeth Graham, Margie Comford and Christine Ristano, my speech therapists, Laura Serine, my occupational therapist, Ryan Cusack, Susan Grant, Kelly Moran, Helen Parker, and Meghan Powell my physical therapists. Powell is a Buckeye like me. The Ohio State University has a lot of living alumni. It seems I am running into them all the time. I should thank Ricky Parker, the ingenious engineer who built many of the things in my home that I use every day, like the bars in my bathrooms and the banister on both sides of my stairs. I would also like to thank Mario Valenti (former Vice President) and Kerry Rice (President) from Upper Loudoun Little League, who gave me the opportunity to be a Little League Head coach in the Fall of 2021. I would also like to thank all of my friends and Brother Knights, who have shown me unbelievable support, given me rides to work, and prayed for me non-stop. I should thank Fathers Gould and Heisler of St. Francis de Sales Roman Catholic Parish for their constant prayers and encouragement. Penultimately, I would like to thank Kim Smith, who used to work for me, for giving me rides to the office. I am truly blessed to have friends like these. Finally, I would like to thank my family – who have been rock solid through this entire ordeal.

Second, I wish to thank those responsible for this book. First, thanks to my friend Jason E. Bartolomei who encouraged me to write this book. His son, Isaac, put my index together and read the entire book (over and over) in doing so. Jason, Kelly, and John Byrnes (Kelly's Dad) read the chapters as I completed them. Second, Janet Box-Steffensmeier, William Patchak, Brian Pollins, Pat McDonald, Ryan Sweeney, and Wesley Wood read the completed manuscript. I needed that help as I was deathly afraid of sending an error-filled manuscript to my publishers. Many on the list were looking for a way to help, and they found it!

Third, I would like to thank all the folks at Bookmarketeers for their support and great ideas. Special thanks to Casey White, who was my entre into the world of book publishing, and a fantastic book marketer; my project managers Eminey Gullmaz, Chris Matthew, and Jack Hudson, Anne Quinn, and Paul Thomson, my editors. And Alan Berry, the Head of Writing and Production for Bookmarketeers.

Table of Contents

CHAPTER 1 AS IT HAPPENED 13

CHAPTER 2 WHAT I WAS 24

CHAPTER 3 AUGUST, AND THE MONTHS THEREAFTER............ 62

CHAPTER 4 COACH KEVIN 91

CHAPTER 5 THE LAND OF FALLING TREES 144

CHAPTER 6 THE DAILY GRIND 170

CHAPTER 7 THE 4 LESSONS 194

CONCLUSION 208

REFERENCES.. 219

INDEX 223

List of Figures

Figure 1: Family and Work Web vii
Figure 2: College Football Stadiums.. 50
Figure 3: Effects of Aphasia 60
Figure 4: My Therapists 90
Figure 5: A Game Lineup 143
Figure 6: Our Game Schedule.. 143
Figure 7: Accomplishments 169
Figure 8: My Bedroom.. 193
Figure 9: The 4 Lessons 197

CHAPTER 1
AS IT HAPPENED

In this chapter, there is a timeline of my very first days as a stroke survivor, including a funny story about receiving Last Rites. There is also a technical understanding of my strokes (I actually had two). Plus, I plan on getting back (most) of the skills I have lost by the time I turn 50 in 2024.

I will start by detailing my stokes. It turns out that one of my two strokes was particularly devastating.

Here is a timeline of the incident (all dates are 2020, that wonderful year):

26 August

~20:00[1] I was on our couch watching the Yankee game after a long day at work. We always got (and still get) Major League Baseball Extra Innings, so I can follow the Yankees though I am (very) out of the market. I rarely got to sit still, as we shall see, but when I did, I would watch the Yankees.

I think Timmy really enjoys watching the games, too (not so much Ryan, Matty, and Kelly, who was the captain of her high

---

[1] All times in this book are in military time.

school gymnastics team and, generally, does not like a sport if there is a ball involved).

I did not ice my knee that night but frequently I would ice my left knee. I tore my left patellar tendon in 2009 playing basketball. There is a funny story about that and how pride comes before the fall. I was at Ryan's last basketball practice of the season (he was 4), and they had a little competition: The dads raced the kids in lay-ups. The kids, with little basketballs, had to make lay-ups at the near free-throw line, and the dads, with a regulation ball, had to dribble the length of the court and make a lay-up at the far end – we all started at the baseline. I felt pretty good (for not having played in five years) after my first lay-up, and after watching other Dads dribble off their feet or with two hands, I decided on my second lay-up, I would show off and dunk. Dunking was something I could do when I was 18, but I had not really tried it after that; I could still palm the basketball. Anyway, for my second layup, I tried to jump high. It was at that moment, in front of a gym full of people, that I tore my patellar tendon, and my left kneecap was in the middle of my quadriceps. I must have gone five feet in the air and landed, with a whack, on the small of my back. My back hurt much worse than my knee. The grown-ups stopped, but the kids kept going. That became my first ride in an ambulance, and I was in a full leg brace for two months.

I complained of not feeling well and wanting to go to bed. My speech became slurred, and I tried to get up and fell back on the couch. My speech got worse, and I tried to get up again and fell to the floor. At this point, Ryan came in, and my wife called 911. An ambulance took me to INOVA Cornwall in Leesburg, Virginia. It arrived fast, and was a remarkably short ride (I think the lights, sirens, and time of day all helped). I remember the paramedics coming and the ride in the ambulance. My wife followed the ambulance to the hospital. The boys stayed home; it was probably scary. There was no telling at that point how much our lives would change, but you can use us as an example – strokes change lives.

22:30 Was when a doctor administered the tPA (Tissue Plasminogen Activator). I wondered if I would be better off if this was administered sooner, but they wanted to be sure I was having a stroke. That said, I was definitely within the 3-hour window for the tPA. I still remember the shot and being in the Emergency Room. They did a CAT scan when I arrived and did not see a stroke even though I had symptoms. Then they did a spinal tap, which I remember, to rule out any bleeding in my brain before giving me lots of medicine. At this point, I was awake, able to speak clearly enough to be understood, and I remember.

~23:00, They transferred me to INOVA Loudoun ICU. My wife, Kelly, was not allowed inside. I also have no recollection of this or events of the next few days and have had to rely on a timeline from Kelly, whose life was changing too. She was not allowed in both because the doctors needed to work, and because of COVID regulations. Without COVID, she still would not have been allowed in.

27 August

09:30 My wife talked to a nurse who said I was alert and oriented. My speech was only slightly slurred. The nurse could understand me, though I have no recollection of talking to him. I was, at that point, waiting for an magnetic resonance image (ing) (MRI) and to see the neurologist. I have spent a lot of time waiting for neurologists. Kelly arrived at the hospital during visiting hours and got onto my floor, but they would not let her in to see me. Kelly has no idea what my speech was like at this point compared to what it was like a few days later after they took me off the vent (I pulled it out).

~16:00 Kelly talked to the ICU doctor, Dr. Lee. She reported a delay in my speech, but I could be understood. Funny, these are the last words I would say. Some test results were back, and all were negative (CT, heart, neck arteries, lungs). I had uncoordinated movements, but my strength was good on both the right and the left (this would remain true the whole time and is still true). The doctor said my impairment as a result of the stroke could get worse for up to 3 days, and it did. He was very right, unfortunately. They planned to move me to the main part of the hospital after 23:00 and get neurological and physical therapy evaluations.

23:00 The ICU nurse called Kelly and said I fell getting out of bed. I was trying to leave and, somehow, understood that a nightmare was unfolding. The nurse told Kelly that I was trying to get up because I vomited. Kelly suspects this was when I had the second stroke, but it could have been any time after 20:00 on 26 August, and when the MRI came back on 30 August. The nurse told Kelly she saw me in the doorway and told me to stay in bed, and she was putting on the PPE when I fell. I guess she could not get to me fast enough. After this, they started strapping me down in the bed so I could not get up. I continued to try; I was a big-time flight risk. The nurse also thought I might have hit my head when I fell, so they ordered a new CAT and MRI. They would have CAT results soon, and MRI results in the morning.

Also at that time, 23:00, the nurse called Kelly back. They got the CAT results and could see the Right Cerebellar stroke. It was large and there was swelling on my brain stem. They were going to transfer me to the neurological ICU at INOVA Fairfax right away. They had not done the MRI yet.

28 August

01:00 The nurse calls Kelly again, and the ambulance is taking too long, so they are putting me in a helicopter to INOVA Fairfax. I do not remember, at all, the helicopter ride, but it was, apparently, quite costly; the helicopter company tried to bill us $40,000.

This calls to mind another helicopter ride I do not remember (because I did not take it). I was in Iraq in 2006, and the Commander of Multi-National Coalition – Iraq (MNC-I), LTG Peter Chiarelli, offered to let me fly with him to Anbar Province to brief the Marines there on a key piece of analysis on which I was working. I said no thanks because I was slated to go home that day. Timmy was due and I did not want to miss the birth. I always regretted not going on that helicopter ride because many Marines, I think, could have been saved by my analysis. Chiarelli later put on a fourth star and became Vice Chairman of the Army. I ended up, among other things, making the Front Page of the New York Times with that analysis, but that is a story we will get to in the next chapter.

13:30 Kelly, a rule follower, arrived for visiting hours. I had the drain in, but only a small amount of fluid was draining. I was sedated, but my blood pressure was quite good, and I could follow commands, though the sedation made it hard to wake me up. The breathing tube was still in.

15:30 Kelly talked to the attending doctor and neurosurgeon. The doctor, brilliantly, said it was a massive stroke. He saw both scans, and it would not have shown up on the first scan because it was done so soon after symptoms. He was concerned that the drain was not working well even though it was in a good position and that I might need surgery. The neurosurgeon said he wanted to keep watching, that I did not need to have a lot of fluid drain as long as I was not deteriorating. They said Kelly would have to wait for the neurological and stroke team evaluation to get a prognosis, which she never got. I am the wrong kind of doctor, but I can say it was very serious, and I was fighting for my life. So, at no point did I see a bright light. Maybe I did and do not remember.

When Kelly got home, she decided to email our Pastor, Fr. Gould, because of the possibility of a major neurosurgery. Kelly wanted to make sure he knew what was going on in the worst case. Fr. Gould called Kelly about 30 minutes later and asked, "Has he been anointed yet? I am going right now." Kelly warned him about COVID protocols, he probably would not get in. It was not easy, and he called her back a few times to try to get her to tell the nurse to let him in. (They did not care what Kelly said). He eventually made it in to see me.

Father Gould, showed up after visiting hours and had to talk his way into the hospital (despite wearing a collar). This shows you how serious my condition was; there was a real chance I was going to die. With Last Rites, I have now had six of the seven Sacraments of the Catholic Church (I am missing Holy Orders and I probably will not get those, so I will not get any new sacraments as long as I live).

29 August

Kelly called several times overnight, and there was no change.

13:30 Kelly arrived for visiting hours. I had pulled out the vent tube on my own and tried to get out of bed. I was still trying to leave. I was breathing fine, so they reduced my sedative and started an anti-anxiety medication. They also increased my restraints. I do not remember being restrained, but I am certain the restraints made me feel confined (more than I was). The drain was still in and working. I was able to respond to Kelly by nodding, but I was very out of it. The doctor said that the impact of a stroke could peak anywhere from one to five days afterward, so they would watch me for two more days. Any sign of deterioration, and they would do the surgery. They were still looking for the cause; they never found one. I still do not know, definitively, what caused my stroke.

Fun fact: the cause for about 1/4 of all strokes, including mine, is unknown. For me, a Doctor at Hopkins came the closest to nailing down a cause, and it looked like a blood clot from my leg (or my heart) and traveled to my brain – a freak occurrence that can happen to anyone. Unlucky for me, odd, because I have always had good luck and have a shamrock tattooed to my left biceps. At any rate, what caused my strokes has been, and will continue to be, far less important than my recovery.

30 August

When Kelly called in the morning, they told her I pulled out the drain overnight and tried to pull out the IV. The drain did not need to go back in. I was still trying to leave. They had stopped the sedative, but I was still sleepy, likely because of the swelling. I was on a hypertonic solution to reduce the swelling. They put in an order for an MRI but had not been called down yet. I was able to have ice chips and apple sauce with my medication.

I did have a stroke, two in fact. Here is the promised technical understanding, from a 30 August CAT scan of my head.

"TECHNIQUE: A CT angiogram of the neck and intracranial arterial circulation was obtained with IV contrast. A contrast-enhanced head CT was performed at the conclusion of the procedure.

Maximum intensity projection, multiplanar rendering was performed. The patient received an intravenous injection of Visipaque 320, 85 cc.

Any proximal internal carotid artery narrowing was determined utilizing the distal internal carotid artery as a reference, similar to the NASCET methodology.

The following dose reduction techniques were utilized: automated exposure control and/or adjustment of the mA and/or KV according to patient size, and the use of an iterative reconstruction technique.

Findings:

The great vessels of the neck originate from the aortic arch.

The right common carotid artery is patent. There is no stenosis of the proximal right internal carotid artery based on NASCET criteria. The more distal cervical right internal carotid artery is patent. The intracranial right internal carotid artery is patent.

The left common carotid artery is patent. There is no stenosis of the proximal left internal carotid artery based on NASCET criteria. The more distal cervical left internal carotid artery is patent. The intracranial left internal carotid artery is patent.

The vertebral arteries are patent. Both the right and left vertebral arteries are patent in the neck. Both the intracranial vertebral arteries are patent.

The basilar artery is normal in caliber.

Duplicated left superior cerebellar artery is noted.

The proximal visualized portions of the anterior cerebral, middle cerebral and posterior cerebral arteries are patent.

No cerebral aneurysm is seen.

No arterial dissection is seen.

For those, like me, who do not speak the medical language, the above means I had one very bad stroke.

31 August

When Kelly arrived for visiting hours, I did not have restraints on and was not on sedatives. I was very calm and more alert. I was able to respond to some questions. My speech varied from clear at times to very difficult to understand. I was also confused. I knew I was in the hospital and had had a stroke. I thought they had transferred me to a hospital in New York, where I am from. Later on, I was more sleepy and harder to understand. We were still waiting for the MRI and CAT scan. They thought they might need to put the drain back in. I finally got the MRI later that day.

1 September

Kelly talked to the nurse and the physician's assistant when she arrived at the hospital. They had MRI results and could now say it was two strokes. My neurological examinations were okay, and I was still sleepy. So, they started me on Lipitor, Heparin (blood thinner), and Seroquel (sleep). I was able to eat with help. The speech therapist and occupational therapist were going to evaluate me. I have seen a lot of speech and occupational therapists since then. They were still looking for the cause, in vain. They were able to eliminate Afib, and neck (vascular), and had sent out blood work for a clotting and genetic workup.

2 September

They were moving me to an Intermediate ICU. I would see an occupational and a physical therapist that day and have a swallow test, and they would schedule a TEE test (A transesophageal echocardiogram) of my heart. I was able to eat a small amount of lunch. I gave Kelly some questions for the doctor at this point, but I really do not remember: How much of the impairment is due to medication, and how much is due to stroke? What is the expected recovery? Good questions. I also said I was having trouble eating and drinking, but it was hard for her to understand what I was describing. At this point, my speech was complicated and I seemed to struggle just to get words out. I was evaluated by speech, physical, and occupational therapists that day.

Whatever the medicalese, the main effects of my strokes were to rob me of my power of speech, they destroyed my balance (which is why I had a wheelchair), and I should say here I have to do everything slower now. It is not clear to me if the doctors knew these effects in September 2020. Probably, I am not the first person to come around with these types of strokes. These symptoms are, simply, too common.

3 September

Acute rehab was recommended, but I needed to wait for a bed to open up. Kelly also checked our insurance, which was to loom large in those early days. There were no other changes. I still do not remember any of this.

4 September

Kelly got some information about Encompass, an in-patient health care provider, which I will expand upon in Chapter 3. I went there afterward and stayed for about a month. I saw the cardiologist again. The results of the TEE test showed a small PFO, a hole between the left and right sides of my heart. This was likely the cause of the stroke. They recommended a heart monitor after I finished rehab. They ruled out clots in the lungs and legs.

5 September

I was transferred to Encompass in-patient care, and I remember getting there. It was a Saturday, and I had a television in my room. There was a lot of commotion outside my room, and it was not easy to sleep that night. Nurses kept coming into my room. Thus starts my in-patient experience, which I remember well, and will write about in detail in Chapter 3.

CHAPTER 2

WHAT I WAS

This chapter details what I was at the time of my strokes; I was many things to many people. In fact, the stress of this all is thought, by Kelly, to have caused my strokes. I fail to see how stress can cause my type of stroke, but be that as it may, there is no doubt my life before was stressful. I plan to shed some activities to decrease the stress in my life. Some of this will come naturally as our kids age out of things; for example, I will not coach Little League Baseball once my boys age out, which is soon. (I wonder what I will do with all the accumulated stuff). It turns out, I am not that far off.

Work [2]

I was, and am, a member of the Senior National Intelligence Service (SNIS) – which roughly means I am equivalent to a Brigadier General. I became a SNIS in 2017, owing to an intense process of competition for which I had to prepare a (about) 15-

---

[2] I found out on Wednesday March 23, 2022, that I was being placed on Administrative Leave to May 31, 2022. At which time I will medically retire from the Federal Government if I pass (fail) a United States Office of Personnel Management (OPM) exam. I think they take qualification for medical retirement seriously, and act like it is a good deal. I opted not to change the book because I will still be a Federal Employee at the time of the manuscript's completion.

page file. While I will always be a SNIS[3], there is much about my job I have lost – I think all because of my inability to talk. This is one area where my affliction has had a huge effect. It is appropriate here to talk a little about my naked ambition. I was about as ambitious as you can imagine, wanting to make Senior Executive by the time I was 40 (I was 43 when I made it). Ambition has taken a back seat to survival now. I will know I am back when I get ambitious again, but I plan on tempering my ambition. My circumstance has provided needed perspective.

It might be easiest to do this chronologically, for a typical workday. Typically, I would get up at 05:00. I would start most days with about a 40-mile drive to the office. I would shower at work most days and put on my suit (which I had to wear) in the locker room. Since COVID I shower and put on my suit at home. Both present their own challenges for me, and I will deal with showering and putting on a suit below. I used to get to my desk around 07:30. In the COVID world I used to get to my desk around 08:00.

I was a Group Chief with about 30 employees I would regularly mentor. We also had a lot (easily 10+) of projects going on, and I was running one massive, center-wide project in which I enlisted the interest of the National Counterterrorism Center (NCTC) Front Office. Both the internal (10+) projects and the massive center-wide project required me to talk to lots of people. That is all over now. I am no longer a Group Chief (since about 15 DEC 2021), my new title is Senior Advisor, and my portfolio of projects was reduced to one project. However, I do still try to

---

[3] You get a 6% raise and a parking spot and must report all financial transactions in your family over $1,000. There are a host of other rules you must follow too – it turns out SNIS membership is not as great as I thought it was. Nobody thinks so.

mentor employees (a SNIS imperative), my center-wide project ended. On May 31, 2022, I will enter a whole new reality where I do not have any people or projects as I enter retirement.

I was a trusted member of the Directorate Leadership Team, which got the President's Daily Brief (PDB), and was 'read on' to a lot of programs. We would regularly strategize, plot really, with Directorate Leadership about positioning in NCTC. I no longer get the PDB (though it is doubtful I would get it now because we have had a Full Leadership Team which we did not have when I was getting the PDB, and the current Acting Lead of my Group does not get it). I have most of the clearances, they tend to be sticky, and I am not called on to strategize, though I do have some ideas. As Senior Advisor, I am part of the Directorate Front Office team; though it is not clear how trusted I am.

The remaining big components of my day, which I do not do anymore, are interviews and phone calls. In the past, I would field 10-20 phone calls a day (from around the government about our projects). I would also make about ten phone calls a day on behalf of our projects. That has ended. Not only do I not have projects to talk about but (owing to my current condition), I cannot talk on the phone. Finally, I was a regular member of Interview Panels (despite not having any under-represented demographic characteristics; I am a White Male). Importantly, Government Interview Panelists all ask a question. I have not been on a panel since my strokes, and we will see when I get on one again.

I used to work in excess of 40 hours a week, or more than 80 hours a pay period (which are biweekly). Since returning I was working four eight-ish hour days a week, though I was advocating to go five days a week. Importantly, all of my doctors and therapists thought I could do it, so did Kelly, and I really wanted to try.' It is worth noting that when I went back to work (at the end of March 2021) I started by only working 5 hours a couple of days a week and have steadily added days and time.

No doubt I fell off a lot after my strokes, but I want to conclude by reiterating how wonderful my Leadership and Office have been throughout this ordeal. My bosses at DSOP, Kulika Frazier and Damon Stevens, were very supportive of me and bent over backward to make my life at work as easy as possible. However, I would be remiss if I here did not mention the support of the entire Directorate of Strategic and Operational Planning (DSOP) – which was truly eye-watering.

Coaching

I will excruciatingly detail my most recent coaching experience in Chapter 4 (which I really enjoyed). Here I will focus on my coaching philosophy and what I hope to teach the kids because this has changed (some would say for the better) 180 degrees since August 2020. I will also talk about the key role my son Ryan played in all of this. All told, I coached thirty teams over more than a decade. Twenty-seven of those teams were baseball; three were basketball. I only coached Timmy in basketball (who was/is a good point guard). I have accumulated a great deal of baseball knowledge (and stuff) over the years. I hope to pass both on. Stuff includes about five dozen baseballs (of two types), small balls (golf ball size), six tees (I only have three sons), three sets of catchers gear, about ten batting helmets, two Zeps meant for the ends of bats to measure a bunch of things (google it), a bevy of baseball accouterments (like batting gloves and donuts,) 5+ gloves (did you know infielders and outfielders have different gloves?), a dozen, or so, tennis balls and dozens of, so-called, heavy balls, and two nets. This does not count my considerable Wiffleball collection. Our garage is overflowing, but the good news is my sons use all this stuff, and yet we buy more as they grow.

I still remember telling a friend, Jason, who I thanked in the introduction, that I would never coach my sons in sports. I was too busy. Boy, was I wrong? I simply did not trust anyone else to do a good job with my kids and took it all on myself. Father still knows best, and I coach my kids one-on-one these days, and I have also had my fill of parents and 'Bobby's' ever-changing schedule – which a head coach of a team needs to keep tabs on. Bobby is a made-up kid; it could be anyone.

I was a win-at-all-costs head coach who wanted to teach the kids so they could perform on the field. So, in this sense coaching the District All Stars, Travel Baseball, or the Middle School Team (all baseball), all of which I did, was perfect for me. Moreover, I believed, and still believe, all coaches are like this, particularly if they are coaching their own sons. I was dismissive of anybody who believed differently. Since my strokes, I care much less about everything, including winning, and coach for the love of the game and to teach the kids, and parents, something about it. If they learn one, or two, things, it is good enough for me now.

I cannot understate the magnitude of this change – it is huge. Even now, as I write it, I am in disbelief. I even wanted to win in Fall Little League baseball, where the score does not count, and offensive teams are limited to 5 runs in a half-inning. I should say I was the same way in basketball, where I taught to win.

My eldest son Ryan played a key role in this, my former obsession, and all the while, I looked for things that would benefit all players to cover my tracks. Ryan probably does not know it. I started with coaching Ryan in Tee Ball in 2011, and it was my perception that he needed my help to succeed. If I was the head coach of his team, I could put him in a position to be successful. My obsession really played in All Stars, Travel, and Middle School baseball, where I would give Ryan opportunities to play key positions and gain experience. I set up the entire Middle School baseball team to give Ryan a leg up. A great example of this is that I nested the middle school team under the high school team to make Ryan known to the High School Coach. What Father would not do this for his son? It turns out he did not need me; being a left-handed pitcher was enough. I prayed hard for a left-handed pitcher before Ryan was born.

Well, if I did it for Ryan, I had to do it for Timmy and Matty. This is how I accumulated 30 teams over more than a decade. Slippery slope, indeed, and it is all over. I never intended to coach in the Spring of 2022, but I did want to umpire (with my sons). I cannot umpire yet but will as soon as I can.

Academia

I was a published author, I still am, and a reviewer for academic journals. I do not do the latter anymore, though that has more to do with kids than strokes. In this section, I will detail my academic publication history and explain the academic review process. Then I will drive the point about kids and reviews home by telling a funny story about my kids and my newspaper subscriptions (there is an inverse relationship). This all was an important part of my life until I turned 30. The change was not because of the strokes and does not have to do with my inability to talk, or any of my other ailments, but is so important to me, I have to tell it. It turns out Academia (and I was going to become an

Academic for the longest time, maybe my entire 20s) is not the meritocracy I thought it was.

Just like every other profession, getting a job, or getting ahead, in academia can be about who you know (and I figured this out in a most unusual way). For the longest time, I thought academia, with its double-blind review process, was a meritocracy. That is, you would get ahead if you scored a bunch of major publications in a short period of time (I did, as you shall see). At least, being a State school kid, I hoped so. I was better than those Harvard kids, right? Well, I got birthed into the Academia-is-not-a-meritocracy school when a member of my Dissertation Committee tried to place me at Harvard, because they had a friend there. It would have been a good placement, but not well earned. It ended up not mattering because 9/11 changed my life, like so many others, and I felt called to work for the government.

I digress. 11 September 2001 is very special to me. My cousin, Alphonse Niedermeyer (google him), was one of the Port Authority Police Officers killed in the Twin Towers on that day. Al was a bona fide hero before 9/11. In fact, he was commended by the mayor (Dinkins) in 1993 for diving into the water when a US Airways flight skidded off the runway at LaGuardia Airport. Al is the reason I decided to work for the government. After 9/11/2001, esoteric academic papers became less important to me, and I decided to forego academia and apply my skills to the terrorist problem. It is fitting that I landed at the National Counterterrorism Center. I have wondered, in the months since August 2020, if I would be as well treated by an academic organization as I have been by the government. Probably not, though I maintain the best job in the world is a tenured professor (if you do not break any laws, you can do whatever you want). Suffice it to say, I know a lot about the Ivory Tower.

I did have quite a few academic publications. In 2003, in the Journal of Conflict Resolution, I published a chapter of my Dissertation after I had a major statistical breakthrough. In "The Severity of Interstate Disputes: Are Dyadic Capability Preponderances Really More Pacific?" I showed that pairs of states view each other's power through the prism of their interest similarity. This makes intuitive sense (NATO) but flies in the face of the established literature. The statistical breakthrough I had was being able to estimate an interaction effect (multiply two variables together, in my case, capability and interest similarity) in a sample selection model. That statistical breakthrough, though it seems trivial, unlocked my whole dissertation.

In 2004, I published three articles in the Encyclopedia of Social Science Research Methods. "Heteroskedasticity" is non-constant error variance, and the opposite is required to derive the Ordinary Least Squares estimator. "Regression Coefficient" is estimated in Ordinary Least Squares Regression, and any two variables will exhibit "Regression to the Mean." I used Shaquille O'Neal's Field Goal and Free Throw percentage to illustrate. Also in 2004, with Paul Fritz, I published two articles on the Balance of Power Theory. In both, "Jumping on the Bandwagon: An Interest-Based Explanation for Great Power Alliances" in the Journal of Politics and in "The (De)Limitations of Balance of Power Theory" in International Interactions, we showed, empirically, that states ally based on interests, not to balance power.

In 2005, Yoav Gortzak, Yoram Haftel, and I put the lie to Offense-Defense Theory (ODT) and showed it had little to no explanatory power when compared with other systematic explanations for war. There is more to the story than that. When I opened the journal with that article were photocopies of the Negative Binomial, Poisson, and Normal Distributions. Systemic wars, our dependent variable, are rare events that explain the Negative Binomial and Poisson Distributions. Both are used to estimate event counts. A photocopy of the Normal Distribution was there because I used that to test the statistical significance of event occurrences, the Negative Binomial distribution – rare events. It turns out Systemic Wars follow a moving average process, and I had to code a so-called "Poisson Exponentially Weighted Moving Average" (or PEWMA for short) Model. This is noteworthy because I used that model to make the Front Page of the New York Times, and I briefed some very high-level Pentagon Officials (think Rumsfeld) on Augustus Poisson, who famously remarked 'life was only good for doing mathematics and teaching mathematics.' He, and his quote, were on the slides that were briefed to Government and military leadership. That quote was simply too good to pass up.

The PEWMA model was a pain in the neck to code, and I got help from the author of that model. Also, in 2005 Omar Khesk and I published "The Similarity of States: Using S to Compute Dyadic Interest Similarity" in Conflict Management and Peace Science. We computed an Interest Similarity Score for every pair of states from 1816 on and wrote a handy statistical program, which we made available, to estimate it. Also in 2005, I published "The Assessment of Non-Physical Human Factors" in the International Council on Systems Engineering Insight Journal. Based on my early work at the Joint Warfare Analysis Center (JWAC), this article gave a listing of social science research methods that could be applied (and I later applied) to interstate and internal conflict.

In 2007 Pat McDonald[4] and I published "The Achilles' Heel of Liberal IR Theory? Globalization and International Conflict in the pre-World War One Era" in World Politics. In that article, we showed that free trade, in an era that is routinely held up as an example of Great Power conflict during globalization, was an era of great protectionism as there were a lot of non-tariff barriers to trade put up by the Great Powers. Pat is one of my best friends, and we shopped that article around for a while before it found a home at World Politics. In 2012, Brock Edwards and I published "The Intelligence Communities Global Posture." In Studies in Intelligence. Brock, also one of my best friends, and I showed readers the posture of the Intelligence Community based on a classified study we did. All told, I was perfect – every paper I sent to a journal eventually got published, a rare accomplishment.

Finally, there is this book, which is under contract and should be published in 2023.

I have tremendous insight into the academic review process because I interned at a major political science journal, The American Journal of Politics (AJPS), near the end of graduate school. The academic review process is double-blind. This means the Author does not know who the Reviewers are, and the Reviewers do not know who the Author is. Typically, when a

---

[4] Pat and I got Ph.D.s in Political Science at the Ohio State University (OSU). Pat is my best friend from graduate school. I could say a lot about OSU, perhaps a full books' worth, but I will only make 4 comments here. First, I enjoyed my time at OSU immensely. Second, I worked, for the longest time, in the Polemetrics Laboratory for Herbert Weisberg. Third, Brian Pollins was the Chair of my dissertation committee, which also included Janet Box-Steffensmeier and Randall Schweller (Pollins and Box-Steffensmeier read this manuscript, so did Pat). Finally, I was the first methods fellow for Box- Steffensmeier. In that way, I was a trailblazer.

paper arrives at a Journal, it is assigned to 3 Reviewers, who do not know each other and do not know the Author. Reviewers are assigned based on their subject matter expertise, and you are most likely to be assigned by a Journal Editor if you have recently published an article in that Journal. The paper's bibliography also provides fertile ground for Reviewer selection, and you are more likely to review if you have done so recently. It is for this reason, and the first, that Reviewers are 'sticky,' that is, the more you do it, the more you do it. If you do not submit papers to Journals (like me) and have not recently reviewed for them (again, like me), you are unlikely to get asked to review. Just as well for me now as I really do not have the time and am not familiar with the literature.

About 80% of papers get 'rejected,' that is, all 3 Reviewers agree the paper is not right for the Journal. The other 20% get invited to 'Revise and Resubmit,' Papers almost never get outright accepted. Typically, 2 of the 3 Reviewers (and the Journal Editor) must see enough promise in the paper to recommend a revision. There is no timetable for the revision, but a month to 6 weeks is reasonable, and the authors of the paper make the changes suggested by the Reviewers, and any by the Editor and submit a letter detailing the changes and counterarguing the Reviews. The revised paper, and this letter, determine whether a paper is 'Accepted' for publication or 'Rejected.' It is possible that a paper will go out for a second round of Reviews. If a paper is accepted, it is about a year's wait before it gets published; such is the waiting line at Academic Journals.

For my papers, when I was invited to 'revise and resubmit,' I was careful to address every point raised by the Reviewers and, especially, the Editor. I tended to write very long letters (10+ pages, single-spaced) and was praised by Editors for my thoroughness. The Journal Editors really appreciated that, and in this sense, my time as an intern at AJPS was golden – I knew, or felt I knew, what Editors wanted.

Well, I really do not have the time to write, or review, now because of a full-time job doing something else, and I have three sons. I tell a funny story to illustrate the effect of children. Before we had any, I subscribed to three newspapers (The New York Times, The Washington Post, and USA Today – for the excellent sports section). I would read all three every day. When we had Ryan, I shed one paper, I do not remember which, and when we had Timmy, I shed another. Finally, when we had Matty, I shed the third. I was out of time and did not read newspapers anymore. It is funny how having kids restrains your time, or at least mine. I certainly would read more if I stayed in Academia. I used to subscribe to, and read, about 12 academic Journals. I am down to 2 now (International Security and Foreign Affairs, they were both relevant to my former job).

I did not even mention books. Before kids, I would read a book a week and spend upwards of 10 hours a week looking for books. I now read about a book a month and tend to read what everyone else (in my field, I still do not read the best-selling novels) is reading. I also now really tend to focus on specific topics for books that interest me. Oddly, to this point, I have rarely read a fiction book (they never really interested me).

Knight

In this section, I will first talk a little about how the Knights of Columbus (K of C) is organized, and then I will move on to discuss my role in them – in particular as an Officer and through various programs, which I will detail. I am a 4th Degree Member (the highest Degree) and a particularly prized insurance member. Kelly and I have the Knights life Insurance, which is pricey, but since the profits go to support a host of charitable activities, we view our premium as part of our tithe. I was very active in the K of C, and it is one of the things I will pare back in my future life.

The K of C is global; they are in the United States and many countries worldwide. The Catholic fraternal service order was founded by Father Michael J. McGivney[5] on March 29, 1882. Membership is limited to practicing Catholic men, which I am. My mother, a Great Lady, encouraged me to join the Knights 'when I settled down.' I 'Settled Down' not long after I got married in 2004. The organization was founded as a mutual benefit society for working-class and immigrant Catholics in the United States. It has grown to support refugee relief, Catholic education, local parishes and dioceses, and global Catholic social and political causes, such as: opposition to same-sex marriage and abortion. It is also an Insurance Company. It's a wholly-owned insurance company, one of the largest in the world, underwrites more than two million insurance contracts, totaling more than $100 billion of life insurance in force. It has the highest possible rating.

There are two ways to understand how the K of C is organized – by membership and by Councils. As far as membership goes, there are 4 Degrees in the United States, and I am a 4th Degree Member. The 1st degree of the order is charity. New members get initiated into the 1st Degree. This is very important, both because membership is the lifeblood of the Order and because I was on the team that conferred the 1st Degree. The second degree is unity, and 1st Degree members are eligible. The

---

[5] Fr. McGivney has been Beatified and needs one more confirmed miracle to become a Saint. Father McGivney, Pray For Us!

3rd Degree is fraternity and is generally accompanied by a test. Only 2nd Degree members are eligible. The 4th Degree, in the United States, is patriotism, and only 3rd Degree Members are eligible. The 4th Degree is organized into Assemblies that have their own Officers and organization. The 4th Degree is significant because they form color guards, which are often the most visible arm of the Knights, to attend important civic and church events. If you have seen a Knight, he was probably in a tuxedo and was probably a 4th Degree Member.

The other way to understand the organization of the K of C is by Councils. Each Parish, generally, has a Council, and it is the basic building block of the Knights. Councils have Officers (I was one) headed by the Grand Knight, who runs the Council (a significant job) and runs all programs in which their members (including me) participate. Councils also have Insurance Agents; I may want to become an Insurance Agent when I retire. They try to sell services to members. Each Insurance Agent typically services multiple Councils. Councils are Organized into Districts (which typically have 6-8 Councils each), and Districts are organized, again in the United States, into States. The Supreme Council sits over the states and the International Organizations and is the highest-level organization. Each level has its own slate of Officers, who, typically, serve one-year terms and are 'voted in' by members. This excludes the Financial Secretary (I was one) appointed by the Supreme Council for a three-year term.

I was very active in the K of C and was both an Officer (at times) and participated in a boatload of programs. As I mentioned, this is one thing I am looking to decrease going forward. I was a Recorder for Council #7812 (Holy Trinity Council in King George, Virginia) in 2007 and 2009. The Recorder takes notes of all meetings and is an Officer 'voted in' by the members of the

Council. I was also the Financial Secretary for Council #11136, at St. Francis de Sales Parish, from 2010-2013. The Supreme Council appoints Financial Secretaries for three-year terms by the Supreme Council. The Financial Secretary position is a lot of work, about 10 hours per week, but it is a great way to meet people, and I met some great people. I decided to relinquish my Officer position. Typically, the Financial Secretary progresses through the Officer ranks and eventually becomes the Grand Knight of the Council. It is also worth noting here that Members refer to each other as "Worthy Brother." I have never known the reason for this.

I participated in many, too many to fully list, K of C Programs. As a sample:

I, annually, participated in the Free Throw contest (which I participated in again this year, and Timmy won his age group). For kids 14 and under, they shoot free throws, and the Council winner advances to the District, and so on. Timmy is an 80-90% free throw shooter and typically wins his age group in the Council and advances to districts (where it is a little bit of a crapshoot). The age cut off is 1 January, and Timmy benefits from being born on 2 January.

Every month our Council hosts a Pancake Breakfast for the Parish, and I used to help clean up (after eating my fill of pancakes). I also made the boys clean up, they enjoyed it... I think it was the chemicals. I do not think I will do this anymore; I would struggle to clean up, and I prefer to eat in private now. This is, for sure, one thing that will change.

Our Council also monthly gathers food for a local food pantry. We have given the Food Pantry well over 2 tons of non-perishable goods. I would participate, in the past, in two ways. First, I would hand out bags, after Mass, (the boys also handed out bags and were very effective – who could refuse a bag from a kid?) to Parishioners as they left the Church. Second, I would pack the trailer when the Parishioners brought back the food. We still participate and contribute food liberally. I could see handing out bags and, of course, contributing food but not packing the trailer, which I would not be any good at now, in the future.

Our Council participates with various other Northern Virginia Parishes in an annual Car Raffle. I participated in the past by stuffing envelopes full of Raffle Tickets (which we mailed to every family in the Parish). I could see, in the future, returning to envelop stuffing (it is an important fundraiser for the Parish). We, of course bought tickets, though it is noteworthy that no one from our Parish has ever won a car. Maybe next year.

I participated on the team that conferred the 1st Degree to new members of the Knights. This was a heavy lift, as I had to memorize my lines. I played the Financial Secretary, which I was in real life. This has changed somewhat in recent times as the degrees are now on CD, and people do not have to remember their lines anymore. It is a shame, as there should be some pain in the degrees. Funny, I still remember my lines and those of others.

Penultimately, I would participate in various projects around the Church (like the annual picnic and putting up and taking down the Nativity). Going forward, I will have to pick my projects wisely, as I can no longer do a lot of physical labor. I did park cars this year at the Loudoun County Fair – on my birthday to boot.

Finally, I would attend monthly Council meetings. Council meetings are important because you get an update on all the programs that are happening and a plea to participate. The meetings started with a Rosary, and the meeting itself lasted about an hour. These meetings got crowded out because of my busy extracurricular schedule. I do not envision returning in the next decade because there are many other ways to discover what is happening, though the Group Rosary is powerful. I would need a ride if I participated in the monthly meetings.

Husband and Father

Hundreds of times a day, you probably take it for granted (take it from me: DO NOT); you talk to your spouse and kids. I do not right now, and it is very frustrating. I mostly text to them these days. This is the way people communicate now, particularly the kids, who always seem to be attached to their phones (at least mine are) to communicate. It is difficult to say if I would be texting this much if I never had strokes, but I miss talking to (yelling at) my kids and whispering sweet nothings to Kelly. In this section, I will first talk about how I used to give verbal guidance to my kids (like discipline), and then I will speak of the family group text. Kelly set it up. Then I will discuss about what it was like to talk to Kelly. I will conclude this section by going over the various topics (we have already covered some ground) I have texted Ryan.

Boys need a lot of guidance and coaching. It is difficult to say how often I talked to my kids, multiple times a day, but that is all over. I used to leave an encouraging note on the kitchen table for them when I went to work. The kids sleep forever. (I still do, and I often text too - things like Cape Diem! and the like. I will also tell them to move the laundry forward, we are forever doing laundry). Now, I will see something and not be able to verbalize a response, but I think it. It is quite frustrating because I cannot text fast enough. I feel boys need their father. This has definitely been one major change since my strokes, and I am looking forward to getting it back. I think I will.

In her infinite wisdom, Kelly set up a family group text that included me near Christmas 2021 (23 December 2021, to be exact). Others mostly use the text to coordinate rides, which is very important, but I tend to use it to send long messages on various subjects (either something I see or something relevant from my past). I use the group text about once a day, and it is great for me. Plus, as I mentioned, this is how people receive information now, for better or worse, so I think it works out just fine. It is a bit of a counterfactual to hypothesize what life would be like if I had not had the strokes, Kelly probably still sets up the group text, but I would not use it as often, or for the kinds of things I use it for now.

I have taken to texting the boys about the previous night's Yankees game. I try to include a fact, or two, that no one knows, this is how I keep the texts fresh. I wonder what I will do when the baseball season ends?

Kelly was always a shy, quiet person and I was a bit louder. I think she was smitten with my sarcastic sense of humor. Well, I still think those things, like before. I just do not say them (and often, they happen so quickly, I cannot write them down). The silence between us is deafening, though I do talk to her more than anybody else and think that my voice will come back with her before anyone else. Suffice it to say, if you love someone, you should tell them now because you do not know when a freak accident could take away your ability to do so. This is definitely one area that has changed and I, very much, want to get it back.

Ryan is at an age, 17, where he needs both a lot of guidance and is inseparable from his phone. I have texted him about a variety of important topics (I had 'the talk' with him over text, and I texted him a long text on shaving and lots of texts on driving), topics from my past that he needs to know about (my friend Matt, who we will meet later in this chapter and my parents, his grandparents, spectacular end, which I will include also) and esoteric topics (like how I became a fan of my favorite sports teams, below, or how I started my baseball card collection, also in this chapter, below). I think this method is superior for him because there is a written record to which he can refer, and, probably, the method of delivery (texts) fits with his life right now. I think I would send texts for most things, maybe not 'the talk,' where I probably set a record.

Fandom

My strokes have definitely not affected my fandom. In fact, my inability to yell at the television is almost certainly good for me, and my family probably appreciates it. Generally, nowadays, I watch games I tape. This way, you can fast-forward the commercials, and you can watch football on fast-forward because every play is replayed. You can watch baseball on fast-forward because the sport is so slow on television.

I break all the rules. Generally, New Yorkers, the downstate type, are not college sports fans. I hypothesize why below and think I am right. But I am a fan of college sports, and always have been. The other way I break the rules is by affiliation. Generally, New Yorkers are fans of teams in 'quadruples' aligned by television networks. Thus, you are a fan of the Rangers, Giants, Yankees, and Knicks. They were all on the Madison Square Garden Network and are all Manhattan teams. Or you are a fan of the Islanders, Jets, Mets, and Nets. They are all teams that were NOT on the Madison Square Garden Network, usually Sports Channel, and are all Long Island teams. As we shall see, I am a fan of the Islanders, Jets, Yankees, and Buckeyes. I do not like

Professional basketball, but if I had to pick, I would select the Nets. I was a fan of the Nets, and watching them regularly when Drazen Petrovich was dominating the League. It helped me the Nets were on 'free TV' (Channel 9).

Yankees

I do not remember exactly when I became a Yankees fan, and it is not related to the strokes; it was a gradual thing. But it happened when I was about 6 or 7. The Yankees were on WPIX 11 in New York, and Phil Rizzuto did the color commentary. He had a host of play-by-play announcers he worked with. I thought he was very funny. He had many stories about his playing days; he won the AL MVP in 1950, and about Yogi Berra, with whom he was a lifelong friend. He is probably more responsible for me becoming a Yankees fan than anyone. I guess I also wanted to be different from my parents. The Yankees also won more games, than any other team, in the 1980s, but they never made the playoffs. There was a good chance they would win every time they were on WPIX, and that helped. I still watch the Yankees, and sometimes I keep score. The only way my strokes and my inability to talk has affected me is that I cannot yell at the television, which I used to do with alarming frequency. I think my family appreciates that I do not yell anymore, but I can assure them and you, I am yelling on the inside.

Soon I was on the hunt for Yankee baseball cards. Don Mattingly was my hero, and I have a lot of his cards. When I was 10, in 1984, Mattingly was great and won the batting title and AL MVP. He won the batting title over his teammate, Dave Winfield. Mattingly was also a gold glove first baseman and the Captain of the New York Yankees. Around 1987 he started to have back problems. They plagued him throughout the latter part of his career, when he was a shell of himself, and forced him to retire in 1995. As a Yankee, he never won a playoff series while Mattingly was playing for them. The 1995 Division Series against Seattle is classic. They lost in what would be Mattingly's last games. In a cruel irony, the Yankees won the World Series the next year, 1996, with Seattle's First Baseman. I could write forever about Mattingly, but I will not.

Anyway, I watched every inning I could on the television and listened on the radio when I could not watch them. My parents were Mets fans, as many former Brooklyn Dodgers fans were. The Mets were meant to be a replacement for the Dodgers when the Dodgers moved to Los Angeles, but they never really lived up. The Mets were on channel 9 WOR in New York, and my parents had pretty much every game, even Spring Training games, on the Television. So, it is important to know that only about 50 games were on 9 or 11, so a game being televised on 'free TV' was an event.

It was not long before I started listening to the Yankees on the radio. I used to listen and hang out in the backyard with our dog, Rusty. John Sterling did the games back then, as now. He used to do the games back then with Michael Kaye. Now Kaye is on YES. I listened to the entire 1998 season, when they won 125 games, on the radio. I can name the entire team roster. It helped that they were winning. They won the World Series in 1996, 1998, 1999, and 2000. They lost the World Series in 2001 in one of the greatest injustices in the world. The entire country was rooting for them. I listened from 1999 forward, but not as much. In 1998, I was in Ohio and used to sit in my car in the parking lot and listen to the Yankees. My car radio was strong enough and this was before baseball was on the internet.

Ironically, as baseball became more available on the internet, I listened less and less, another thing that fell away as I became busier. A baseball game, a Yankees baseball game, is ideal to have on in the background while you are doing something else, and it is fun to listen to the games and score them. In fact, when I retire, one of my goals is to follow the Yankees around for a season – going to all 162, or however many there are then, games.

Islanders

I am a rabid fan of the New York Islanders and have been since I was a kid. I still watch their games on NHL Center Ice. In this section, I describe their glory years when I became a fan. My inability to talk has, again, only affected my ability to yell at the television, much to my family's delight. Hockey is a simple game and they mess it up all the time.

The Islanders won four Stanley Cups in a row in the early 80s, when I was a kid, and are considered the last dynasty in major North American sports. They also won 19 playoff series in a row, a record. They lost in the Stanley Cup finals, in the "drive for five" in 1983, to the Wayne Gretzky Edmonton Oilers.

They had some great players on those teams who are in the Hall of Fame. Foremost among them is Mike Bossy, who is considered the greatest natural goal scorer to ever play. He holds many records. Bossy had lung cancer and died in 2022. He hurt his back and had to retire in 1989. Criminal. Many people, me included, feel that trading for Butch Goring, who does the Islanders color commentary now, was the final piece. I know the entire lineup. Billy Smith was the goalie and is considered by many to be the greatest goalie ever. Denis Potvin was the key defenseman, and was, without a doubt, the most outstanding defenseman to ever play the game. Al Arbour was the coach. He has the second most coaching wins of all time and is considered one of the game's greatest coaches. Bill Torrey, who always wore bowties, was the General Manager. Arbour and Torrey have both passed away, but they left many fine memories.

The Islanders were not on 'free TV,' and I used to go over to my friend Ed Scott's house to watch with him and his father. His Dad drove a delivery truck for Pepsi, and Ed's house was always well stocked with soda, which I drank, liberally.

I grew up very close to the Nassau Coliseum, where the Islanders played. It was nicknamed Fort Never Lose. I kept, keep, thinking they would return to prominence. They almost did in the late 80s/early 90s with Pat LaFontaine and Patrick Flatley. I used to listen to the radio and shoot pucks, or balls in the street, on a net I had. Sometimes I would shoot with Ed.

I still remember going to the Stanley Cup victory parades down Hempstead Turnpike, very near where I lived. I thought they would win every year. Boy, was I spoiled?

Jets

It is odd to be a really big fan of a bad team, but I am a huge fan of the Jets, and my strokes have really had no effect on that, except I cannot yell at the television anymore. With the Jets, there is a lot of yelling. This is a moribund franchise that last won (well only won) the Super Bowl in 1969. They are the author of more disastrous moments, like the butt fumble, than great moments, but my fandom stretches way back, and the Jets had training camp very near my home growing up. That is why I am a fan—proximity rules.

Where do I start? Well, the Jets had training camp, as I was growing up, near my house at Hofstra University. They go to Upstate New York now. I used to go to training camp nearly every day. It was great to be that close to all the players. You could literally reach out and touch them, and I got hundreds of autographs over the years. Football teams have training camps at universities because the players stay in the dorms as they have to practice twice a day, "two a days" The Jets players were no different. In fact, the best time to get autographs was when the players walked from the dorms to the practice field. Training camp was also good for scouting various plays and players. I would get a good sense of who was on the first team and what plays they would run. As Yogi Berra said, I observed a lot by watching.

I would watch every game with my friend, Bob Villatore, who now lives in San Francisco, and his dad, Bob. Occasionally, Bob's grandmother would join us. Bob Sr. was a Levittown[6] lifer who went to Division Avenue High School, like Bob and I. He would regale us with stories of 1969 when everybody won: the Jets, Mets, even Division Avenue High School football won the Long Island championship, the Rutgers Cup, that year.

I would paint my face green and white before going to their house to watch the games, which were like an event. I would also eat a lot of pistachios, which are green nuts, while watching the games.

---

[6] I grew up in Levittown, New York. The world's first Suburb. I could write forever about Levittown, but there is a great documentary about Levittown, called, "Wonderland," you should watch – it is really about America.

As I said, the highlights have been few and far between, but there have been some; two stick out. First, in 1986, they won 10 consecutive games, and they were picked against by Paul McGuire every game. He worked for NBC and would pick the games on the pregame show. I still remember the great players on that team. They lost in the first round of the playoffs that year. Second, there was one great, record-setting, game on September 21, 1986, where the hated Dan Marino and the Jets quarterback, Ken O'Brien, had a classic duel. The Jets won in overtime 51-45, and my favorite player, Wesley Walker, a receiver who was legally blind, had a big day and caught four touchdown passes.

Buckeyes

I am an enormous Ohio State sports fan (mostly football). In fact, my spirits (still) rise and fall with the fate of the football Buckeyes. I care less about the men's basketball team and even less about the other sports – though the men's volleyball team is good, and I have a soft spot for wrestling. Like me, if you are sick, I will encourage you to check out elevenwarriors.com for great coverage of Ohio State sports (mostly football). They have great tee shirts on the website.

I was always a college sports fan but really did not have a favorite team; college sports are not that big in New York. As an aside, it is interesting to think if there is an inverse relationship between professional teams and college sports. At least, I think that was what was happening in downstate New York. I think college sports got drowned out by professional sports. "Upstate" New York tends to have more college sports fans. Anyway, as with the other teams, my inability to talk has only affected my ability to yell at the television.

Growing up in college football, I liked teams that ran the wishbone, like Oklahoma, Nebraska, and the Service Academies. In college basketball, I liked St. John's. They were good in the early to middle 1980s, and some famous players went there, such as Chris Mullin and Mark Jackson. Lou Carnesecca was the basketball team's coach. He too was/is famous least of all because he wore a different loud sweater every game. He won various games, and in 1985 3/4 of the Final Four (Villanova, Georgetown, and St. John's) came from the Big East.

Anyway, I had offers from Indiana and Columbia for graduate school and picked Ohio State because they had a superior football team. I got season tickets, by myself, to football my first year (and then with friends thereafter).

Funny Ohio State football story, I lost my parking spot when they 'improved' the Stadium in the quest for the largest college football stadium. Ohio Stadium currently seats just over 102,000, but it is not the biggest college football stadium:

RANK	SCHOOL	STADIUM	CAPACITY[7]
1	Michigan	Michigan Stadium (Ann Arbor, Mich).	107,601
2	Penn State	Beaver Stadium (University Park, Pa).	106,572
3	Ohio State	Ohio Stadium (Columbus, Ohio)	102,780
4	Texas A&M	Kyle Field (College Station, Texas)	102,733
5	Tennessee	Neyland Stadium (Knoxville, Tenn).	102,455
6	LSU	Tiger Stadium (Baton Rouge, La).	102,321
7	Alabama	Bryant-Denny Stadium (Tuscaloosa, Ala).	101,821

Figure 2: College Football Stadiums

---

[7] The 25 biggest college football stadiums in the country | NCAA.com, accessed 1 February 2022.

They made it bigger, but I do not think they made it better… too clever by half. To make it bigger, they took several steps, including lowering the field, removing the track (that was around the football field), and putting in permanent stands to close the horseshoe. That was a good thing because the temporary seats were like an erector set and scary. I sat, way up, in them once. They also replaced the turf with artificial grass. You do not have to mow it, but it has been shown to cause cancer.

Anyway, the Stadium expanded into the parking lot, and I lost my prized parking spot. It turns out that Ohio State, being as large as a city, has many cars, and parking is tight and difficult.

Basketball tickets were easier to get, and I went with my friends that first year. The basketball team played in St. John Arena my first three years, and the Schottenstein Center thereafter. 'The Schott' was built because it seated more, but I still prefer St. John Arena.

Card Collecting

I have a massive baseball (and some football and hockey) card collection. All told, I think it is worth as much as a new car. I still remember when I got my first pack of baseball cards. It was 1981, and I was home sick. My mother bought me a pack of baseball cards, and I was hooked. I could not read yet, I was in kindergarten, and I tabbed the Seattle Mariners as the Devil's team (I was right, see the 1995 playoff series against the Yankees) because they had a pitchfork logo. This section will first talk about some of my baseball card sets (Topps) and star cards. Then I will talk about my massive doubles from the 1980s and some of my other sets from other companies (such as Fleer, Donruss, and

Score). I will conclude by talking about my star football cards, which I am willing to trade for baseball cards I need. I am eager to do this; my football cards are worth about a thousand dollars in trade. My strokes have not affected my baseball card collecting. In fact, at the baseball card show I went to in December 2021, I bought some 1969 Topps cards – I was putting that set together when I had my strokes. My cards are Timmy's – he will take good care of them. Funny story, when he was four, he asked me for them because "I never took them down to play with."

To start with, you must understand two things. First, all cards are produced by companies. Topps, which has the longest-running tradition, has been producing baseball cards since 1952. Second, I aim to own all the Topps Sets before I die. There are other companies that produce cards, and this speaks to our second key point. The market for cards became oversaturated in the 1980s, driving card values way down. It turns out I was not the only one collecting. Part of the saturation was because of other companies entering the market. I collected Fleer, Score, and Donruss. I also collected Bowman, which started to make cards again in 1990, and I have that set and 1991 as well. Bowman last produced cards in 1955. And as we shall see, I have several of their most noteworthy cards from that early period, including the crown jewel of my collection. But I did not collect several others, most notably Upper Deck. With those two things out of the way, we can move forward. The headline of my collection, without a doubt, is that I have every Topps baseball card from 1970 onwards. I was putting together the 1969 Topps baseball card set at the time of my strokes. My goal is to get the sets all the way back to 1952 when Topps started producing baseball cards, but the 50s and 60s are pricey and might drive me out of the market. We will see, I am willing to leverage my other cards to get these sets, and this may be my saving grace.

I have several other star cards which deserve mention, including the Crown Jewel of my collection – a 1951 Bowman Mickey Mantle. The first card ever made of him (remember, Topps did not start producing baseball cards until 1952), my father got it for my 8th birthday at a garage sale for $100. In its present condition, it is worth about $4,000 in cash and $6,000 in trade.[8] My other notable cards include 1951 and 1952 Phil Rizzuto Bowmans. The 1951 version is famous. Painted the year after he won the American League Most Valuable Player Award (AL MVP), it features him in a joyful pose reaching up for a ball (he played Shortstop). I also have 1954 and 1957 Yogi Berra cards. The 1957 version is noteworthy because it mentions, on the back, that he won American League MVPs in 1951, 1954, and 1955. Can you imagine what a Catcher with 3 MVPs to his name would be worth today? Lastly, I have a 1969 Mickey Mantle as part of my collection of 1969 baseball cards. It is the last card of him ever made (he retired in Spring Training, 1969). So, I have bookend Mantles.

I have a little bit more baseball card education to share. For a variety of reasons, Mickey Mantle cards are worth the most (the 1952 Topps Mickey Mantle, in mint (pristine) condition, tends to sell for about $1,000,000). Pete Rose and Nolan Ryan are also worth a lot. Also, you should know that rookie cards are worth about 5x-10x what later cards of the same player are worth. In fact, if you are in the market for complete sets (like me), rookie cards in a set typically drive up the set's value. Cost is my major driver now. If anyone is looking to get rid of sets, or knows someone who is, let me know.

---

[8] That is another very real thing to know. Generally, you can get around 150% of cash value in trade.

I have a lot of other sets, and doubles, from the 1980s. As far as sets go, I have every Fleer[9] set of baseball cards from 1983 to 1991. I have the Score sets from 1990, when they started, to 1992. Finally, I have every Donruss[10] baseball card set from 1983 to 1991. I also have about thousands of doubles from the 1980s, when I tended to buy packs of cards and put sets together. Some of my doubles from 1982 and 1983 are probably worth something, but most of my doubles are, unfortunately, worthless (even in trade). This is a shame because I am willing to trade to meet my ultimate goal – it would be very cost-effective. You will note I stopped collecting around 1992 when I started dating Kelly and all my excess income went to her (not baseball cards). After we were married, filling in those missing sets, as well as the current year's set, made very good presents for birthdays and Christmas.

It is also worth mentioning I kept a book, which I still have, of star baseball cards from the 1970s, 1980s, and 1990s. The first player in that book is Don Mattingly (see above).

I have a lot of Football Cards from the 1980s, and unlike baseball cards of the same era, they are worth something, and I am willing to trade them. Apart from sets, which I have, I also have:

- A 1984 Dan Marino and 4 1985 Dan Marino action cards

- A 1983 Lawrence Taylor in action card[11]

- 2 1983 Jim McMahon cards

---

[9] A Canadian manufacturer.

[10] Another Canadian Manufacturer.

[11] The 1984 Marino card is his rookie card. In a crying shame now, Taylor and Marino were often pasted to dart boards by me because I really hated them – being a Jets fan. I ruined about $500 worth of cards.

- 2 1984 John Elway cards (his rookie)
- A 1983 Joe Montana card and a Montana in action card from that same year
- A 1982 Ronnie Lott card and a Lott in action from that same year
- 3 1986 Reggie White cards (his rookie)
- 3 1986 Steve Young cards (his rookie)
- A 1984 Eric Dickerson
- A 1984 Darrell Green
- 2 1984 Russ Grimms

I mention Green and Grimm on the list because one can often get more money for a card in a player's home market, and I am in the home market for Green and Grimm. It is worth noting that this geographic arbitrage is a way to make money when you sell (or trade) cards.

Finally, I have all the hockey card sets from 1983 to 1991. My hockey cards were manufactured by Topps and by O-Pee-Chee, a Canadian manufacturer of hockey cards. The listing of football cards excludes the untold thousands I have in Gretzky, Yzerman, and Bossy cards. I bet I have a lot because I have numerous hockey card doubles, though the 1985 Gretzky probably found its way to my dartboard.

So, I have one more card for each of the stars listed above, and I have one for everybody else. It is what I did with my money in the baseball off-season and putting together those sets was good off-season fun. I would get money. I delivered newspapers from 1985 to 1989 and then worked in a delicatessen from 1989 to 1992.

My sports cards mean a lot to me, as they are mementos of my youth and feed my obsessive-compulsive desires. Even now, I often look through them when I am feeling depressed and have already earmarked certain boxes of cards to go through when I retire.

Mourner

I have lost three really significant people in my life, and they have taught me to fight. Since I am in the fight of my life now, knowing this and honoring them is super useful. They drive me from the grave. My strokes, and my inability to talk, have not affected my ability to mourn; in fact, I still pray for Matt, and my parents, daily. This section will start with Matt and then move to my parents, Charles and Kathleen, whose spectacular end in 1997 taught me I could do anything.

It is difficult to overstate the importance Matthew James Arroyo has for me. Matt was my friend growing up, and he died (on 21 August 1991) just before what was to be our senior year in High School. During our sophomore year, Matt got sick with Hepatitis; we never knew why. But he ended up having two liver transplants before he ultimately succumbed to the disease. The grace and dignity with which he bore his illness are a real inspiration for me now. He really taught me how to fight, and I fight for him. The fact that he never got married, had kids, or lived long enough to have a stroke really drives me. So before we move on to my parents, I will tell you a little more about Matt, including an amazing story (of which I have a very special memento).

Well, I will not bury the punchline. Growing up, Matt was a huge fan of both Dwight Gooden and Pat LaFontaine. Gooden played for the Mets, Matt's favorite baseball team, and LaFontaine played for the Islanders, Matt's favorite hockey team. Both wore number 16. Amazingly, when we got to High School, Matt was assigned locker 1616. Well, after he died, I had that locker cemented shut so nobody would ever occupy it again. I kept the locker number, which I carry in my wallet. Matt was so significant, in fact, we named our third son after him. Why not the first or second? Well, we really liked the names Ryan, Patrick, Timothy, and Sean. That is why we have a Ryan Patrick and a Timothy Sean.

Matt and I were friends from the time we were five – even though we went to different Elementary Schools – a big divider in Levittown.

Matt's family sat one pew in front of mine at St. Bernard's Roman Catholic Church, and Matt, and I were both part of the gifted and talented program in Levittown and we were all bussed to a special school once a week. I have great stories about the latter; not much interesting happened in church. We knew each other from an early age and quickly discovered we had much in common, including a love for the Islanders and Pat LaFontaine.[12] Matt got to meet LaFontaine (there is a picture of them on p. 80 of my High School Yearbook, which is dedicated to Matt), and Lafontaine sent flowers to Matt's funeral.

---

[12] LaFontaine played for the New York Islanders from 1983 until 1991 (when he was traded, in a deadly blow, for 4 players), to the Buffalo Sabers from 1991 until 1997, and the hated New York Rangers from 1997 until his retirement in 1998, scoring 468 goals and 1,013 points along the way before his career was ended by concussions. His 1.17 points per game (1,013 points over 865 games) is the best among American-born ice hockey players, active or retired. It is worth noting that one of the players Lafontaine was traded for, Benoit Hogue, now lives in the same housing development as my in-laws on Long Island.

My parents, Charles and Kathleen Sweeney, had an amazing end in 1997, which taught me how to deal with adversity. It also led to my engagement to Kelly, who was right there for me the entire time. Significantly, her parents, John and Sue, had me over for dinner every week.

Charles was an abusive alcoholic who smoked four packs of cigarettes a day and died of cancer in 1997. My mother, Kathleen, was basically a Saint, and died in 2009 – but that is far from the most significant fact in her story. In September 1997 my mother put my father, who was rapidly declining, (cancer had metastasized and spread to his brain) into hospice care and promptly had a cerebral aneurism at work. She recovered somewhat and she was driven home. My Uncle Al found her the next morning; he was, fortuitously, coming over to go with my mother to find a permanent place for my father. She was dead and was revived in the ambulance on the way to the hospital.

My mother was in a different hospital than my father, but they were both in intensive care units (ICUs) of their respective hospitals. When this all happened, my brother, Pat, and I were out of town. He was in college in Buffalo, and I was at Ohio State in Graduate School. Significantly, I was living in the dormitory, and my phone had not been hooked up yet. So, I got a frantic message to come home via the Front Desk from my Aunt Carol (who was my Uncle Al's wife). Well, I rushed home, and I gather my brother got the same kind of call because he drove through the night, and, not having a key – broke down the back door to our house. I arrived the next day in chaos. Not only did I find out about my parents, but the back door to the house I grew up in was busted and the dog, Rusty, had peed and crapped all over the house. I later found out that the dog and the house were infested with fleas. The fleas became a running battle for me.

I stayed home, and Pat went back to school. All told, I missed 2 quarters of graduate school. My father died in October, the same night the Yankees lost to the Indians in the ALDS. My Mother graduated from the ICU to the hospital, an in-patient rehabilitation facility, and lived with me at home. You would have had to know her beforehand to know something was wrong. I went back to school in the spring, but my mother had a series of seizures that really degraded her ability. Seizures cause brain damage; she had multiple. We never really figured out why, but the leading possibilities were the metal suture in her head and an allergic reaction to all the medication she was on. I like the latter. There was, and is, no telling how various medications interact with each other. Doctors sure do not know. Ultimately, we found a home for her, and the dog, in Upstate New York – where my brother was. So, we decided to move her to him because I knew I would move from Columbus, OH, after finishing graduate school. It was a real shocker to all that I left Academia behind.

Driving

I will not have too much to say about driving, which is odd since it is one of my highest priorities. Driving was a priority for me because I had to shuttle kids around and commute to work. Plus, I liked it, though I hated traffic (which we have a lot of in Northern Virginia). I used to drive everywhere, but now (see above), I do not drive at all. I used to drive 80 miles round trip to work (living so far away), shuttle the kids around town, and run numerous errands around town. That is all over. I get driven now. Ironically, Ryan has his license, and Timmy will be right behind him. So, by the time I can drive again, I will not need to perform one of my major functions. I do practice driving now about every week in the parking lot of a baseball field I frequent. I wonder if this 'practice' will address the main concern with my driving. The main concern with my driving seems to be with my slowed reaction time; if anybody knows a way to simulate reaction time while driving, we are all ears. As of mid-summer 2022 my reaction time is about .51 seconds, only one thousandth of a second greater than the 'normal' range for my age. Nevertheless, I think the effect of my inability to talk on driving is medium because I cannot talk to police officers or other motorists now.

Conclusion

So, let us take stock. With the help of Figure 3, we can see my Aphasia is only having a middling effect on the big activities of my life. It has fully affected work but has only partially (or, had no effect) on the other aspects of my life – a surprising, good news story! I think a far greater effect has been had by my slowness, which really affects everything (including writing this book). So, my goal to get faster in 2022 is a good one.

Scorecard	Aphasia Have An Effect?		
Work			Full
Knights			Partial
Husband and Father			None
Fandom			
Collecting Cards			
Mourner			
Driving			

Figure 3: Effects of Aphasia

I will end on a hopeful note. I continue to make progress every day (Kelly and I believe, I will get back all the way). In fact, in

Chapter 5, I will detail when I tied my shoes for the first time, cut down a Christmas tree – it is a family tradition, and went to a baseball card show. That all happened, as did many firsts, near the end of 2021. That said, the season of firsts is ending for me, and the season of getting faster is starting. I can now do most things, albeit slowly, which is hard for me because I used to do everything fast. I know I need to get faster at doing things and will focus on that now.

Other good things have happened: I lost 15 pounds, stopped drinking Diet Coke (maybe this caused my stroke, the doctors still do not know), stopped drinking alcohol (not that I drank that much, I mostly drink water these days), stopped chewing gum (which was constant for me), my teeth are much better (I floss twice a day and use mouthwash in the morning, good habits I picked up at Encompass Health, above), am properly thankful, and I think my situation has led one of my son's, Ryan, to find his calling in life. Rest assured, I will keep fighting for every yard with the same type of steely determination my friends and family have known me for. This fight is likely to take years, and with everybody's help, I will win it. Meliora!

For you, Meliora is a Latin word, the motto of my alma mater (The University of Rochester), and perfectly describes what is going on with me. It means, always better… not like I am better than you, but like I am always improving. And, I intend to keep improving for a long time if necessary.

CHAPTER 3
AUGUST, AND THE MONTHS THEREAFTER

Encompass – Beginning the Long Road to Recovery

I was in Encompass Health and Rehabilitation Center of Northern Virginia (hereafter Encompass) from 5 September 2020 to 23 September 2020, and it was the longest three weeks of my life. I will say at the outset (because I will be highly critical of my time at Encompass) that they were consummate professionals, and I would highly recommend them if you, or a loved one, need their services. It was a long three weeks, as we will see in somewhat shocking detail, because I was (mostly) cognizant by this point, and I basically knew what was happening to me. I really wanted to get out of there because of the many indignities I suffered (two of which are recounted below) and the general hell I was living. There was a big difference between weekdays and weekend days. Basically, nothing happened on the weekends. That is how I break up this section. In each part, I first talk about what a typical day entailed, then I go through each day. I first talk about my arrival – which I remember perfectly.

I arrived at Encompass on a Saturday. I remember the ambulance ride to Encompass because it was unusual. I was in the back and strapped down. I should have known what I was in for from my arrival, but I was too far gone (at that point) to make much of a connection. I arrived at about 20:00H and really wanted to sleep but kept getting interrupted by nurses coming to my room. It was a harbinger of things to come. It was here I first met my primary nurse; I did have others. I wish I remembered his name because he had a profound effect on my life, but I do not. I remember he was African American, and seemed, when he talked, to be from one of the Islands (not Jamaica, I would have remembered that). Unfortunately, he was the author of one of the indignities I will mention.

My arrival was unceremonious. I was transferred from the ambulette bed to the hospital bed in Encompass and bundled up, and, as I mentioned, I just wanted to sleep. Part of my interruptions was nurses, or people coming in to offer drinks (juice, water, or iced tea). Encompass was big on drinks; I guess people recovering from strokes do not drink enough. Encompass seemed to be full of people who had strokes, though I think people who suffered other traumatic brain injuries could go there.

A typical day at Encompass began around 06:00H, when one of my several nurses came into my room and helped me get ready. This included going to the bathroom, getting dressed, brushing my teeth and hair, and putting on deodorant. I had a store of clothes in a dresser that Kelly had brought from home: sweatpants, sweatshirts, underwear, tee shirts, and socks – which were problematic, as we will see below. This was very important, because it was 'my' stuff. I wish Kelly had brought some baseball caps; I have 100s. I think better with a baseball cap on, and am, generally, more comfortable wearing one. I have so many because I got a new one with every team I coached. Because the boys were always on my team, they got hats too, and we were overflowing with baseball caps. I was then wheeled out to wait for breakfast, which was served in the dining room, and it started at 07:30 (lunch was also served in the dining room, dinner happened in the room. We filled out a menu, for all three meals, the day before. I will talk about meals below because the dining room was where the full heterogeneity of patients was on display). I was then wheeled from the dining room to my room. The television was put on the channel of my choice and I was given the remote. I watched television until my next event, which was very different Monday through Friday and on the weekends (where my next meal was frequently the next event). And then I was wheeled from event to event. Because I was cognizant, I can say with 100% certainty; it was like being trapped in a horror movie. Typically, Kelly visited daily, around dinnertime, And I went to bed around 20:00H. I had my pillows from home, which was very important, and made me feel, 'normal.' Lights out at Encompass was 22:00H, and, as I mentioned, I was, basically hourly, visited. It is here where I started the unfortunate practice of texting Kelly around 03:00H, or usually after I was interrupted and woken up. Typically, Indignity #1, I was woken up 4-6 times a night by nurses and a variety of other staff (many offering drinks). That was very annoying to me and was the biggest reason I wanted to leave – basically, I did not want to get woken up in the middle of the night anymore. I was also tired of the bright lights on in the hallways outside my room. Yes, you sleep with your eyes closed, but lights have always bothered me.

The tremendous variety at Encompass was on full display in the dining room – where everyone went for breakfast and lunch. Some people were, basically, catatonic and had to be fed. Some people looked normal. I was in the middle. About half the people were in wheelchairs. We always got our meals served to us (as ordered the day before) and always had the table to ourselves, because of COVID restrictions. The cafeteria ran like clockwork, and the staff there were very professional. In fact, I would say the meals were one of the best things about Encompass. You add the efficiency of the staff on top of very tasty meals, and you really have something.

Weekends at Encompass

On weekends, I usually got up at 06:00H and went to bed around 20:00H. The weekends were like the weekdays in that I was visited 4-5 times during the night. Typically, on weekends my engagements would be my meals. For breakfast and lunch, I was wheeled to the dining room. I ate dinner in my room.

As I mentioned, not much happened on the weekend. In fact, I was left one Saturday until 14:00H – which was basically okay. There was good college football on, but I did miss breakfast and lunch that day, and got my medicine late. One similarity between weekends and weekdays at Encompass was the steady drumbeat of my medication – I was on lots. I watched a lot of sports at Encompass on the weekends. For whatever reason, Formula One racing on Sunday morning sticks out. This is odd because I never watched formula one racing at home, though I was familiar with who the top drivers were (Lewis Hamilton).

The neglect on the weekends was another reason why I wanted to leave. Most of the staff (therapists and office staff) were off on the weekends, and Encompass ran on a skeleton crew. A big highlight of the weekends was Kelly, or Kelly and the boys, visiting. Weekend visits tended to be in the afternoon. I do not know if the visiting hours were different on the weekends (from the weekdays, but the boys certainly had more freedom). The boys had to wave at me through the window because of COVID restrictions.

Weekdays at Encompass

Weekdays at Encompass were much busier, and I always got a schedule the day before (I have one of my daily schedules, 21 September 2020, what were you doing that day?) and have based this section on it. I think Encompass was busier on the weekdays because of the influx of therapists and office staff. It must be much harder to find a good parking space on a weekday. At any rate, Monday through Friday was when the action happened there. I remember a feeling of foreboding on Friday afternoons. I saw my primary nurse on weekdays, he also worked on Saturdays, and he generally gave me my medication in the late morning. He is the author of one of my grave indignities, Indignity #2, as among that medication was a shot, I had to get in the stomach. Trust me; you have not lived until you get a shot in the stomach.

I had Physical Therapy (PT) twice a week at Encompass, and I had Aparma Iyer for PT. Encompass had its own gym, and Aparma was noteworthy because she was much smaller than me and was constantly afraid of me falling on her. Aparma, like all therapists at Encompass, I think, came to my room to get me, and she wheeled me, or I wheeled myself, to the gym (which was about 1,500 feet away from my room). Generally, we did exercises designed to get me walking again, I think she would be proud of my progress, but it would not surprise her. PT with her was generally hard, and I often broke into a sweat. I felt like I needed a shower when we were done. PT was also the place I got fitted for my 'permanent' wheelchair, which we still have. I remember there was great difficulty getting me a chair that fit, I have very long legs.

I had Occupational Therapy (OT) twice a week while I was at Encompass, and I had Nicolas Denizli for OT. He was very young, and I got the impression this was his first job. In fact, all of my therapists at Encompass were on the young side. I wonder if Encompass Health, a National Brand, is the first stop for people in their career progression. Nick, as he preferred to be called, came to my room to do OT. He was noteworthy for two related reasons. First, I had my first shower with Nick. I often think of him when I am in the shower now. Showering was, and is, very challenging. Most of the challenge now is that I shower left-handed on the advice of Margie (a Speech Therapist, below), and I also sing in the shower (Chapter 6). Second, Nick helped me get dressed after my showers and did not like my socks, which were very hard to put on (admittedly). Well, I kept the socks; sorry Nick. He is also noteworthy because he had several ingenious gadgets designed to make my life easier. He sent me home with some of them. The one the boys have the most fun with, but I do not use, is a grip to pick things up. Like a giant claw on a stick, it turns out it is also a weapon you can use against your brothers. All of my therapists are listed at the end of this chapter.

I also had Speech Therapy (ST) twice a week at Encompass, with Michele Villarreal. Sometimes Michelle and I would work in my room, sometimes, we would work in the dining room. But she always came to me. Clearly, she also spoke Spanish, I remember wondering if speaking two languages was an advantage for a speech therapist. I still have, and do, many of the things she recommended. Because my speech lags far behind my other skills, her stuff from long ago is still relevant. At Encompass, the big focus of speech therapy was getting my articulation clear enough for others to understand me and/or getting me set up with augmentative communication (the phone app, now the excel extension that I can use to type what I want to say and have it speak for me). Another big thing for Michelle was she did not want me using straws, and I think of her now when I use one. Michelle recommended a swallow test for me. Swallow tests are, literally, that. They test your swallowing; I rode in an ambulette to that test – which was in another building. The driver, and his aide, are noteworthy because of their extreme professionalism. I really liked Michelle because she had an easy way about her.

PT, OT, and ST have become a big part of my life. In this way, Encompass foreshadowed what was going to happen to me. With six appointments and weekly six meals in the dining room, I had a lot of downtime at Encompass – which was mostly filled with watching television in my room. I hate downtime and really wanted to leave Encompass because of it. I guess I thought that I would, magically, have more to do. Well, that has not worked out, and, in this way, Encompass foreshadowed things to come too.

I will conclude by re-iterating that I really wanted to get out of Encompass. I will make two general observations. First, while the therapists (and social workers) were good, the other staff, especially the overnight staff, were not as good. It was difficult to get someone to help me if I needed anything after dinner (unless they visited my room). That said, they did come when I rang the call button. I could only get a shower at times Nick put it in his schedule to help me (I used to shower daily). Some of this could have been that they were short-staffed due to COVID, or it could just be the nature of the job, too many people to see, not enough staff, and no one really wants the overnight shift. Second, Maria, the Social Worker, was excellent and really helped us to get settled at home. Clearly, she had a wealth of experience.

I should finish this section by making two points. First, I started to wonder at Encompass (and have wondered many times since) whether all the therapy really made a difference. I mean, would I just improve with time? I do not know, call this a great counterfactual hypothesis. I really think therapy helps me get better faster. One thing is crystal clear, I did not appreciate, at Encompass, the large role PT, OT, and ST was to play in my life. Second, I really wanted to leave Encompass. Some of this was due to neglect and the indignities I suffered, but, mainly, I wanted to leave because of me. I have never had time for this, and Encompass was the first time I was 'with it' enough to really conceive of what I was missing and what I was.

Coming Home

I vividly remember the trip home – September 23rd, 2020. It was brilliantly sunny outside. I remember leaving Encompass and getting in the car. I was only this happy when my kids were born. It was the first time since my strokes that I rode in a car, let alone the front seat. Kelly drove me, and I think she was nervous because she kept asking how I was. Kelly later told me that my balance was still so bad at this point that every movement of the car shook me to the point she thought I would be car sick. The boys made me a welcome home sign, which I still have and will probably always keep. I came home to a bit of a surprise, and I will start there.

When I first got home, and until the 3rd week of December 2020, I slept in the living room in a hospital bed. I never really thought about where I would sleep at home while I was at Encompass. I guess I thought I would sleep upstairs in my bed, like usual. Foolish. Anyway, sleeping was to get quite interesting, as we shall see. In this section, I talk about my hospital bed, then the heart monitor I had to wear for a month (which only complicated things) and my poor hematologist, then all of my various at home and outpatient therapies, and all of the wonderful gadgets in our house that were put there by Ricky, the engineer. The last thing I will talk about in this section is my speech therapist, Elisabeth Graham, who I started seeing during this period. I conclude with some thoughts about my speech therapist, the hole in my heart, and how unlikely it seemed that I would have the stellar achievements I had near the end of the year. The best way to conceptualize this is that my recovery is slow and will take several years.

Hospital Bed

As I mentioned, the hospital bed was in the living room, on the main floor of our house. We got the hospital bed, which was all set up for me when I arrived home, from a private company recommended by Maria, the Social Worker at Encompass. Judging from when they picked up the bed in December, the company was very professional. At this point, I really struggled to roll over; the destruction from the strokes affected everything. I have always been a stomach sleeper and I got very used to sleeping on my back in the hospital bed (which was only further complicated by the heart monitor I had to wear). Generally, lights out at home in the hospital bed happened around 20:30H, and there were a variety of strange noises I had to contend with. The main culprits were the fish tank in our living room and the refrigerator in the adjoining kitchen. The fish tank made no end of guggling noises that I had never heard before, too far away, I guess, being upstairs. The fish tank was practically next to me in the living room. The refrigerator made standard refrigerator noises, but I bet you have never listened to yours in the middle of the night. I am here to tell you that refrigerators make some strange noises in the night.

I should make a special note here of our couch, which was also in the living room. At this point, though I tried, I could not get up and down from our couch. The couch is kind of squishy, and that comfort for normal people was a real problem for me. It quickly became the bane of my existence. I remember sitting on the couch and not being able to get up the day I got home. I eventually mastered the couch long before I moved back upstairs (figure around Halloween).

I had to wear a heart monitor for the cardiologist for 30 consecutive days. The heart monitor was meant to measure any arrhythmias I might have. I wore the monitor on my chest, between my pectoral muscles, and it was related by Bluetooth to a cell phone, which we kept on a small table beside the bed. The cell phone was provided to me. There was/is a company that monitored the readings from my heart monitor and provided 24/7 service. The most unpleasant thing about wearing it was that we had to shave my chest to get the adhesive on the back of the monitor to stick to my chest. I also did not dare roll over in bed with the monitor on, I both did not want to damage it, and I was afraid of getting the wire tangled up and accidentally pulling it out of the monitor. As I mentioned in the Introduction, the cardiologist wanted to surgically close my PFO. Heart surgery seemed a little invasive, and if the PFO already caused a stroke, would it cause another one? I was saved by Dr. Llinas, the neurologist from Johns Hopkins University and Hospital, who advised against the surgery. I like to think he was affected by my argument that surgically closing the hole was like lighting birthday cake candles with a flamethrower. Dr. Geloo was my cardiologist, and visiting him was a little like, if you give a mouse a cookie… he was very professional, but surgeons are going to want to perform surgery.

We searched, for a long time, for a cause of my strokes. Perhaps we were asking why. Perhaps we were hoping to find a cause we could prevent in the future. Our quest led Dr. Tuwiner, my neurologist, to prescribe that I see Dr. Firestone, a hematologist. I guess there can be markers in the blood of strokes. She, Dr. Firestone, looked and looked but did not find anything. She nearly bled me dry in the process. I really appreciated her efforts, even though they were in vain. All the while, I was 'sleeping' in the hospital bed. The cardiologist and hematologist happened at the same time – the holiday season of 2020.

Home Therapy

Encompass previewed a lot, and as I mentioned, it presaged how therapy was going to be a large part of my life. During this period, I had PT, OT, and ST at home. When I came home in September, I pretty much immediately started doing the same three therapies at home – all three came to my home at defined times. All three also took my blood pressure before and (for PT) after. I got used to getting my blood pressure taken. They wanted to assure themselves that I was not under any stress. I had physical therapy (PT) with Erica and Megan, the PT Assistant. Their main focus was getting me to walk. They had a series of useful drills to do (using cones in Megan's magic backpack). I did a lot of heel-to-toe walking (like a sobriety test) and walked around the island in my kitchen. We also practiced on the stairs in my house. I have become quite good at going up and down stairs.

I had occupational therapy with Krista; she was, by far, my favorite. We, too, focused on getting me to walk, but the drills were somewhat different. Krista introduced me to putty (I would hunt for beads or coins, for her to work on strength and dexterity), she also had me use the kitchen utensils, she measured my wheelchair for our bathroom (It is really a commode), and shower upstairs, and came up with several ingenious solutions that I still use. Foremost among these is a u-shaped bar for my bed. It slides underneath the mattress and sticks out above it such that the handle part of it is above the mattress and available for me to use. It is still there and probably will always be there. It has been a while since I was in the wheelchair, but I use the bar every morning.

I had in-home speech therapy with Laurel. She ended before PT and OT, and I got the distinct impression she did not know what to do with me. While I got the feeling from all my other therapists that they had worked with a lot of people like me, I did not get that impression from her. Generally, we would do activities in her binder designed to get me to talk – drills where I would read, or repeat, specific words. We got to the end of the book, and the therapy ended. It was near then that I started seeing Elisabeth Graham (see below).

Before we get to Elisabeth, who had a large effect on my life, I should talk about the Engineer, Ricky, because many of the things the PT and the OT were doing were dependent on Ricky installing various gadgets in my house. Ricky, we also found through Maria, the excellent Social Worker at Encompass. She referred us to a different company in Leesburg, and they gave Kelly Ricky's number. All told, Ricky put in my pricey wheelchair ramp (he drove through the night to get it), the bars in my bathrooms, and the banisters on my stairs. The ramp has long since come down (It is in a pile beneath our deck. It has been replaced by stairs with railings for me to hold on to). Though I do not need the ramp anymore, I will probably always use the bars and banisters. I cannot overstate the profound effect Ricky had on my life. He should be proud; he helps a lot of people.

I first saw Elisabeth Graham, of the Speech-Language and Literacy Center, in November 2020. I saw her for speech therapy (ST), but she proved to be much more. I both saw her at her house, from which she ran her business, and virtually. We did several activities designed to get me to speak, like reading from lists of multi-syllable (4, 5, and 6 syllable) words and the Interactive Metronome (IM). The IM is really a system and a computer program. You had to follow a beat, which you could set from a control panel, with either your hands or your feet. The IM also came with headphones, so you alone could hear the beat. The IM gave you immediate, color-coded feedback if you were late or early to a beat. We also had a regular metronome that I would do on the iPad. I was rhythmically challenged before my strokes (I did not sing and really did not like dancing), and really struggled with the IM. We tracked my progress, or lack thereof, in a spreadsheet. Doing the IM was kind of like eating Brussel Sprouts, you know it is good for you, but you do not like it anyway. The IM people claimed marvelous successes for those that used the system, and I wonder if I am one of their successes. Elisabeth also suggested I do Lumosity.com and track my scores in a spreadsheet. She later suggested that I focus on five specific games, and I gladly did this work. I really liked the games on Lumosity.com, and tracking my scores appealed to my competitive side. I stopped doing Lumosity.com when I stopped seeing Elisabeth ~ 1 June 2021.

I would add something that applies to all therapists - Neuroplasticity - that is, the brain's ability to change and adapt due to experience. All therapists believe in this and have tried to help me develop it by doing things with both sides of my body at the same time. Examples include but are certainly not limited to reading or singing while riding the bike and talking while walking on the treadmill. It is basically trying to get both sides of my brain to work to make up for the part that was damaged by the stroke. There are a million examples, and they apply to every imaginable kind of therapy (including the three flavors I have repeatedly sampled).

Holidays 2020

By the time Thanksgiving rolled around in 2020, we had a lot, much more than most people, for which to be thankful. I was alive, after all. This is despite the fact I was not sleeping particularly well and wearing a heart monitor. We went to Mass (we always go to Mass on Thanksgiving. I mean, who are you thanking?), watched the Macy's Thanksgiving Day parade and football. The Parade is a bucket list item for me. We also ate a lot of Turkey. I used to play football on the Front Lawn of the United States Capitol (with Jake, whose idea it was I write this book). I believe I will play again; all it will take is for the US Air Force to assign Jake to the Washington DC area. I already messed with the assignment process for Jake once, and I suppose I could do it again.

Christmas 2020 was noteworthy for me because of what I could not do. I really struggled to order presents and did not contribute any ideas to the boys' presents. I also could not wrap up the few presents I bought. This changed totally in 2021; not only could I wrap I also got Kelly, and the boys, a lot of presents. I have already started to buy presents for Christmas 2022 and have full lists for Kelly and the boys. I do remember I got a lot of presents in 2020. The present I most used, wore every day, was a pair of sneakers Kelly got me. From Kelly, I also got a handy basket for the front of my walker, which proved quite useful. We also went to Mass, after opening presents – Matty still gets up around 06:00H; he also did this year and will probably do so in 2022. After we got back from Mass, the boys and I watched some basketball. We ate at about 15:30H. If you cannot tell, Christmas is a big deal in the Sweeney household.

I used to stay up on New Year's and watch The Ball drop, but not anymore. Going to see The Ball drop never interested Kelly or me. I also used to drink champagne, but I do not drink alcohol anymore. It is just as well because 1 January is a Holy Day of Obligation – which means Roman Catholics must go to church (it is the feast of the Solemnity of Mary, the Holy Mother of God, one of the oldest feasts in the liturgical calendar). I think on New Year's Day 2023 Timmy and I will go to the Rose Bowl – his birthday is right after Christmas. Going to the Rose Bowl is another bucket list item for me. We will need to find a Catholic church in Pasadena, California. Odd thing, me almost dying has made us (me, in particular) much more likely to spend our money. You cannot take it with you.

Out-Patient Therapy

After that brief detour, we are back to therapy - PT, OT and ST, specifically. In January 2021, I started outpatient therapy at Inova Loudoun Hospital. I remember, initially, not liking the idea of doing out-patient therapy. I was nervous. But, Ryan (PT), Laura (OT), Margie (ST), and the office staff (Heather and Jackie, in particular) made me feel welcome. I have probably, made the greatest progress physically over time, and I owe a lot of that to Ryan Cusack – who was great. Generally, we focused on getting me walking. We did some exercises on the mat to start. We would walk around a track they had in the gym, and did a lot of exercises in, essentially, parallel bars they had there. Then played a walking game, like a scavenger hunt for post-it notes in the gym. I remember two times, near the end, Ryan took me outside to walk – which was great. It really helped that Ryan liked baseball; it gave us something to talk about. My time with Ryan ended in May 2021, (which was a shame, he was great), when he left Inova Loudoun Hospital, but before he left, he recommended I go to Ability Fitness (AF) with Helen Parker. This ended up being a great suggestion.

I went to Ability Fitness, in Leesburg, Virginia, with Helen from 1 June through, basically, the end of 2021. I went to AF twice a week. AF was really a hybrid place – it was both a PT place (Helen really knew her stuff) and a gym for disabled people. Most of the people who went to AF were wheelchair-bound and could talk much better than I. At AF, there are a couple of mats and a lot of gym equipment. Before my strokes, I used to use the elliptical every morning, and I used the elliptical at AF for the first time since my strokes. I cannot tell you how important this was. I also spent a lot of time at AF riding an exercise bike, something I also used to do a lot, and walking on a treadmill. Helen was very into me narrowing my support base when I walked or stood. I still remember this advice and really try to keep my feet close together all the time. I was taught six stretches for my hamstrings (which are tight). I do those stretches every morning. Helen was a real professional who did the Lord's work, and it was really difficult to leave.

Ultimately, I left Ability Fitness near the end of 2021 to try to consolidate my therapies in space (do them all at Inova Loudoun Hospital) and time (it has long been my goal to do all of my therapies on Friday mornings). I saw Kelly Moran at Inova Loudoun Hospital on Friday mornings. She was great too and focused on two things – first, getting my heart rate up (I would wear a heart monitor and walk fast on a treadmill); second, getting me to walk heel to toe. For the latter, I do a lot of resistance walking, that is, have someone try to pull me back when I am walking (with a band around my waste) and walking in the hallway sideways. I have also boxed with her, practiced stairs with her, and did the agility ladder (which we have at home).

I see Laura Serine, at Inova Loudoun Hospital, for OT. I saw her from January 2021 to the end of July 2021, and I started seeing her again around the start of November 2021. Laura has been very concerned with my vision; she is the only therapist to be so concerned. She is right to be concerned. People who have stokes, particularly my kind, often have a sharp decrease in their visual abilities. I have really enjoyed seeing Laura; maybe I just really like OT, and we have done a lot of dexterity games with peg boards; we also have worked on throwing a ball back and forth and have practiced writing, typing, stapling, and using paper clips. There are two other things I would mention with Laura. First, she introduced me to the BITS machine (Bioness Integrated Therapy System). The BITS machine is a large television screen where I find patterns of numbers and letters. I really like this machine, and all of my other therapists at Inova Loudoun Hospital have used it. A typical game is how quickly I can put letters on the screen in alphabetical order by touching them.

Second, Laura is really into me reading. In the first go-around with her, I would read a book and then give a presentation on it. This helped my reading and oral expression. I did presentations on nine books for Laura, generally one every other week. We worked up from me reading my slides aloud, to writing separate notes to read, to trying to present from a general outline rather than reading.

In approximate order, I did Trapped in the War on Terror, by Ian Lustick (whom I know); The Year of the French by Thomas Flanagan; Unbroken, by Laura Hillenbrand; Goodbye to All That, by Robert Graves; Inside the Kingdom, by Robert Lacey; The Looming Tower by Lawrence Wright; Directorate S, by Steven Coll; Unmasking the Islamic State, by Patrick Sookhdeo; and, Chain of Command, by Seymour Hersh. Here is my unedited presentation on Directorate S, so you can see where I was. The book is by Steven Coll, and the presentation was dated 12 February 2021:

A 20 Minute presentation on

Directorate S By Steven Coll

By Kevin Sweeney

- Introduction – Afghanistan in 3 Easy Steps
o Civil War and Conflict
o Drugs and Corruption
o Pakistan
- Order of the Slides
o Whose Who?
o What the US Leadership was doing on 9/11
o US Demands of Afghanistan and Pakistan in the wake of 9/11

- o Ahmed Shah Massoud

- o Coll's Unbelievable Access

- o Why is Afghanistan Taking so Long?

- o Drugs

- o Corruption

- o Iraq

- o Rumsfeldian Delusions

- o Killing Bin Laden

- o The Role of Pakistan

- o Conclusion

- Whose Who? (*I knew, or at least Briefed; Was in this Office on 9/11)

- o Abdullah Abdullah – (AFG) Minister of Foreign Affairs (2001-5), Chief Executive (2014-)

- o Mahmud Ahmed – (ISI) Pakistan Director-General of Inter-Services-Intelligence (1999-2001)

- o Engineer Arif – (AFG) Head of Intelligence Northern Alliance (1994 – 2001) Head of National Directorate of Security (NDS) (2001-4)

- o Cofer Black – (CIA) Director of the Counterterrorism Center (CTC) 1999-2002

- o Richard Blee – (CIA) Chief of ALEC Station 1999-2001, Chief of Kabul Station 2002, Chief of Islamabad Station (2004-5)

- o John Brennan – (CIA) Director of Central Intelligence (2013-17) o Wendy Chamberlin (State) – US Ambassador to Pakistan (2001-2)

o Hilary Clinton – (State) Secretary of State (2009-2013)

o *Mike D'Andrea – (CIA) CTC Director (2006-2015)

o Abdul Dostum – (AFG) Deputy Defense Minister (2003) Vice President (2014-)

o Karl Eikenberry – US Commander in Afghanistan (2005-7), US Ambassador to Afghanistan (2009-11)

o *Michael Flynn – ISAF Intelligence Chief (2009-10)

o Porter Goss – (CIA) Director of Central Intelligence (2004-6)

o Ibraham Haqqani – (AFG) Representative of the Haqqani Network (2001-)

o Richard Holbrooke – (State)US Special Representative for Afghanistan and Pakistan (2009-11)

o Jim Jones – National Security Advisor (2009-10)

o Hamid Karzai – (AFG) Chairman of the Interim Government (2001-2), President of Afghanistan (2002-14)

o Ehsan ul-Haq – (ISI) Pakistan Director-General of Inter-Services-Intelligence (2001-4)

o *Mike Hayden – (CIA) Director of Central Intelligence (2006-9)

o Ashaf Kayani - Pakistan Director-General of Inter-Services-Intelligence (2004-7), Chief of the Army Staff (2007-13)

o Zalmay Khalilzad – (State) US Ambassador to Afghanistan (2003-5) o *Peter Lavoy – (US Various) NIO for South Asia (2007-8), DDNI Analysis (2008-2011), PDASD for Policy (2011-14), Director for South Asia NSC (2015-6)

o Doug Lute – 'War Czar' for POTUS (2007-13), US Ambassador to NATO (2013-7)

o Ahmad Shah Massoud – (AFG) Commander of the Northern Alliance (1996-2001)

o *Stanley McCrystal –JSOC Commander (2003-8), Director Joint Staff (2008-9), Commander ISAF (2009-2010)

o *Mike Mullen – Chairman of the Joint Chiefs of Staff (2007-2011)

o Leon Panetta – (CIA) Director of Central Intelligence (2009-2011)

o *David Petraeus– (CIA) Director of Central Intelligence (2011-2012)

o Amrullah Salah – (AFG) Intel Advisor to Massoud (1997-2001), Head of the National Directorate of Security (NDS) (2004-7)

o Gul Agha Sherzai – (AFG) Governor of Kandahar (1992-94, 2001-3), Governor of Nangarhar (2005-2013)

o George Tenet – (CIA) Director of Central Intelligence (1997-2004)

o Chris Wood – (CIA) Afghan Specialist ODNI (2010), Kabul Station Chief (2011), Director CTC (2015-7)

- What US Leadership was Doing on 9/11

o ALEC Station and CTC (pre 9/11)

- o Blee
- o Black
- o Tenent
- o POTUS = The President
- o VPOTUS = The Vice President
- o SECDEF
- o SECSTATE

- US Demands of Afghanistan and Pakistan in the wake of 9/11

- o Afghanistan
- o Deliver to US authorities all leaders of Al Qaeda hiding in your land.
- o Close all Terrorist Training Camps.
- o Hand over to the US all Terrorists in those Camps.
- o Give the US access to all training camps to ensure they are not operating.
- o Pakistan
- o Stop Al Qaeda at the border, intercept arms shipments, end support to Bin Laden.
- o Give US planes overflight and landing rights. The US should have access to Pakistani Naval bases 'as needed.'
- o Should provide intelligence and immigration records for any Terrorist suspects.
- o Publicly condemn the 9/11 attacks.

o   The ISI should cut off all fuel shipments to the Taliban and block all Pakistani 'volunteers' from fighting in Afghanistan.

o   Should evidence point to Al Qaeda, and should the Taliban continue to harbor Bin Laden Pakistan should break diplomatic relations with the Taliban.

- Ahmed Shah Massoud in a Slide

o   Started by Fighting against the Soviets

o   Commanded the Northern Alliance (who was fighting against the Taliban and Al-Qaeda)

o   Was on The CIA payroll (for nonlethal aid)

o   Was, probably, the US's best hope

o   Was Assassinated 9/9/2001

- Coll's Unbelievable Access

o   NSC

o   Conflict Resolution Cell (Lute, Holbrooke, Michele Flournoy, Chris Wood, David Sedney (Flournoy's Deputy))

o   9/16/2010

o   DCs and PCs (in the White House Situation Room, no less)

o   Demonstrated throughout the Book

o   Classified Meetings, Papers, Products

o   Knows about the District Rubin's secret talks with the Taliban

o   Gives the CIA a Pass for 9/11

- ISI (Inter Services Intelligence Directorate)

o   Seems to know what they are thinking

- o Has their entire Organizational structure
- o Named the book after one of their Directorates
- ○ Even knows what Directorate S is/does
- • Why is Afghanistan Taking so Long?
- o It's Complicated
- o Drugs
- o Corruption in Afghanistan
- o Iraq
- o Rumsfeldian Delusions
- • Drugs
- ○ Poppy production exploded in Helmand Province in 2006
- ○ Cash Crop!
- ○ Suicide Bombings also Increased – Primarily targeting military targets
- ○ The Taliban earned(s) up to $500M annually (from ushr and zakat taxes on the poppy crop)
- • Corruption in Afghanistan
- ○ 3 Types – according to Holbrooke
- ○ High Level- Karzai and his Relatives
- ○ Predatory Theft – Cabinet, dependent on Karzai
- ○ 'Functional' corruption – run of the mill
- ○ Karzai's brother (Ahmed Wali)
- ○ Khalilizad

- Iraq
  - A Competing War
  - Not as much Focus in the Book
- Diverted Focus
  - Central Command, and the Military
  - Personal information
  - Rumsfeldian Delusions
- Who is the Enemy?
  - Taliban had a resurgence starting in 2005/6
  - Strategy Reviews of no Strategy
- Rumsfeld's Delusions
  - The War in Afghanistan is Won!
  - 2007 – Greater Spending on Afghanistan (greater than all other years combined)
- Killing Bin Laden
  - Early March – Panetta first shows Obama a model of the Abbottabad Compound
  - 30 April – Martyrs Day in Pakistan
  - 1 May – Operation Neptune Seal (Navy SEALs) Kill Bin Laden
  - ISI role in Sheltering Bin Laden not known
  - Pakistan probably knew
  - Bin Laden had a large network in Pakistan

- His youngest wife, Amal, gave birth to four kids while in Pakistan
  - The Role of Pakistan
  - Supported the Taliban
  - The ISI supported Lashkar-e-Taiba
  - India, Pakistan, Kashmir
  - Conclusion
  - This Book is a Sequel to Ghost Wars
  - It covers the period from Sept. 2001 to 2016
  - Directorate S Solved (Part of the ISI – responsible for covert actions)
  - We will probably still be fighting in Afghanistan when we are old and grey (Maybe not!)

I have the slides too, if anyone is interested.

In the second iteration, Laura is, again, encouraging me to read – this time for pleasure. This is something I used to do regularly. On her suggestion, right now, I am reading two books – one on Hezbollah for work and one on baseball (that Kelly actually got me for Christmas this year) for pleasure. I got Kelly three books, one she wanted, one she needed, and one, sort of, a gag gift. It is really the first thing I have read for pleasure since the strokes.

I saw Margie Comford at Inova Loudoun Hospital for speech therapy for, basically, the calendar year 2021. Margie and I became friends, and Margie really hit it off with Kelly. Significantly, we chose Margie over Elisabeth because of our desire to consolidate in May 2021. Margie was also very concerned with our insurance, which has a cap on the number of speech therapy sessions I can have annually. It is complex, but basically, because I was double-dipping with Elisabeth, we very quickly approached my cap in the calendar year 2021 and ended up having to take some weeks off.

Margie was the first one to tell me about neuroplasticity – which she was really into. When I did stuff with her, it would often be a 'parallel processing' task designed to get at this exact fact. Margie always also pushed me with probing questions – no matter what we were doing. Unquestionably, this was good for me, but I found it somewhat annoying.

I had very strong emotions with Margie. At times, I felt she and Kelly were teaming up on me and not showing me the proper amount of respect, I am a Senior Executive in their government. With the benefit of hindsight, I realize they were just trying to help me and did not mean, certainly, any disrespect.

I did an unbelievable amount of stuff with Margie – most of it was designed to get me to talk. This included expanding the content of my oral language, speaking fluently, and using expression rather than a flat tone. It would be useless to try to recount all of that here, so I will make four summary points. Probably the longest-lasting three things she suggested were, first, showering left-handed, which I will probably always do. Second, she encouraged me to play the keyboard (we bought one, which we will probably always have) and sing in a choir. I was never that musically inclined, so both things were a stretch for me. I gave up both. Margie was very pro-music as an important way to get me talking again and increase the expression in my voice. Third, Margie, at the end, encouraged me to do the Elevate application. I will probably use this application for a good, long time. Margie was also famous for sending me home with a lot of various papers to practice my oral expression. Ultimately, it ended with Margie because of our desire to consolidate therapies on Friday mornings. Margie could not find a time that worked for us, and I will not bump up against my insurance limit for speech therapies this year – as of 20 February 2022, I am still waiting for a new speech therapist.

All my therapies are listed in Figure 4 on a timeline. If you had issues keeping up – do not worry; it has been challenging for Kelly and me. The figure is convenient, and I referred to it several times while writing this chapter.

Conclusion

I conclude by saying I really failed to appreciate how large a role PT, OT, and ST would play in my life. This was all really previewed for me at Encompass and kept right on rolling along. It is almost like there is a therapy sub-culture out there. I now know all about it. I would also say the end is in sight. Kelly had to fill out her election form for the next school year in February 2022. I encouraged her to go back to work full time, which means she will have to be in the office Monday through Friday, 08:00H - 1630H, which effectively means an end of therapy in September 2022. I will get an answer to my counterfactual at that point. I am concerned about backsliding on various skills and will try to do what my therapists have recommended at home. I can now conceive of how to do about 50% of it.

PT	OT	ST		Date
In Home - Megan	In Home - Krista	In Home - Laurel	Speech Language Literacy Center - Elisabeth	09/28/20
				10/01/20
				11/01/20
				12/01/20
Inova Loudoun - Ryan	Inova Loudoun - Laura			01/01/21
				02/01/21
				03/01/21
				04/01/21
		Inova Loudoun - Margie		05/01/21
				06/01/21
Ability Fitness - Helen				07/01/21
				08/01/21
				09/01/21
				10/01/21
				11/01/21
				12/01/21
				01/01/22
Inova Loudoun - Kelly	Inova Loudoun - Laura			02/01/22
		Inova Loudoun - Christine Risano		03/01/22
				04/01/22
				05/01/22
Inova Loudoun - Meghan				06/01/22
				07/01/22
				08/01/22

Figure 4: My Therapists

CHAPTER 4
COACH KEVIN

It is funny; there was very little evidence of me coaching at work besides seven, or so, team baseball plaques that I kept above my desk... only the head coach got those and only in the Spring.[13] It is almost like I was leading a double life. I would work, then (most days) I would rush home to coach a practice. It started as an obsession to coach Ryan; he needed my help, I perceived, and he was the lefthanded pitcher for whom I prayed. Then it became, well, if I did it for Ryan, I had to do it for Timmy and Matty.

All told, I coached about 30 teams. If that is right, and it is close, twenty-seven of those teams were baseball three were basketball – where I only coached Timmy (who was/is really good). In fact, one of my favorite things in the world is to watch Timmy play basketball. Along the way, I met some great people and learned a lot, and I was always learning. I know a tremendous amount about baseball (my favorite quote, reproduced below, is from a very famous person who said, 'baseball is like Church, many attend, few understand. You should know because it is an

---

[13] All Quotes in this chapter are from four sources: the Ted Williams quotes are from (Williams, various), the Satchel Paige quotes are from (Paige, various), the Yogi Berra quotes are from (Berra, various), all other quotes are from (Plaut 1992). I cite them here, and not below, so as to not make unnecessary clutter and disrupt the flow of the chapter).

integral part of my identity. I coached Little League baseball at every level (Tee Ball to Majors and District All Stars), and I was the very first coach of the Blue Ridge Middle School Baseball Team. I still coach my sons, mostly one on one. And, I have had my fill of parents.

In a very real sense, me being the head coach for the Majors River Bandits, Matty's Fall 2021 Little League team was the culmination of years of experience. I am grateful to Upper Loudoun Little League (ULLL) for giving me the chance – which I took very seriously (see below). I had to keep track of many moving parts. I thoroughly enjoyed coaching. I contacted the team almost daily and have reproduced those communications, with applicable attachments chronologically here:

Kevin Sweeney has sent a message on TeamSnap.

Wednesday, August 12, 2021

All,

Welcome to the ULLL Fall Majors River Bandits! I am happy to be your coach for the fall season. There are also three assistant coaches, my son Ryan Sweeney, Jamie Marsh and Chris Thompson. Ryan plays baseball at Valley, and Jamie and Chris are experienced coaches.

Attached you will find a "Parent Meeting on Paper" and some "Always and Never" rules to share with your players. Please read through both and let me know if you have any questions. I also need to get uniform info to the league right away (by noon Saturday), so please respond below (by noon Friday).

ULLL is ordering one green and one yellow shirt per player. We will get River Bandits hats (which are very cool). Please verify the information below and let me know by Friday at noon if you need to change the size or number. If I do not hear from you, I will assume you are good to go. From the list, it looks like MB will be #1 (M wins because he is the head coaches' son); aside from that, everyone will get their first choice of the number!)

2021 Majors River Bandits Parent Meeting Points

The Prime Objective:

#1 Goal – The boys get better. Fall is NOT about winning games; it is an instructional league.

Expect we will meet three times a week until we 'Fall back' (~ end of September), then once a week thereafter.

I have prepared detailed practice plans around the prime objective.

I will try to reschedule games when they get rained out.

I will write some 'always' and 'never' rules to share with the boys. These rules generally apply equally well in life.

I will share daily baseball quotes on team snap. You can delete these or use them.

Required Volunteers:

I will need a lot of help, please, every family help. If you are going to help in any capacity, you need to fill out a volunteer form:

[web link], expect to do a background check.

Ryan (our oldest, who took over for me last Fall and plays for LVHS) will help at practice and during games (he is excited), my wife Kelly will do Team Snap, and Matty (our youngest), is on this team. This team is a Sweeney family affair and a BIG part of my continued recovery.

Timmy, our middle son, and a rising freshman at LVHS, will help when he can too, but he is running cross country and playing basketball, and has a busy practice schedule.

The home team is responsible for field preparation for games, and we should drag/rake fields after we practice.

I cannot do any of this, you will have to, and Ryan can help.

We will also need a scorekeeper (in Gamechanger), a pitch counter, an adult game coordinator, and 2 additional game coaches.

There are many roles to fill; you need not 'know' baseball.

Me:

If you are not tracking my progress (you are one of the few), I have a little bit of an update for you:

I had 2 strokes in August 2020; one was 'devastating' according to my neurologist, the strokes occurred while I was Managing the Minors River Bandits for ULLL, and a lot of people stepped up to help.

I have been recovering ever since.

I remember all baseball, and this will be my ~11th season coaching at all levels in LL, including All Stars, and travel. So, you are in good (albeit somewhat limited) hands.

These days I am very limited in verbal communication and am about 50% physically, which is a shame because it is these two skills (precisely) that are required for coaching baseball. That said, I have several other attractive qualities; foremost among these is that I properly understand that each day is a gift, and I tend to inspire people... maybe I will inspire your sons. I am also near 100% cognitively and understand the written word. These days I can, generally, do most things. It just takes me longer.

This team is a big, huge, part of my recovery.

Medical Release Forms:

All Players must fill out a Medical Release Form

[web link]

Please print it out, fill it in, and give me the hard copy now. I will keep these with me all season

The League, properly, also takes concussions seriously, and there are more forms for that.

COVID Regulations:

Nothing heard, though I have asked the question.

More to follow.

Trophies:

Please give Kelly $10 by 20 August 2021.

My plan for this is every player will get a participation trophy, and the coaches will vote on an MVP, Cy Young, and 4 Gold Gloves – the winners will get additional trophies[14].

We want to make this a memorable experience for the boys.

---

[14] This was not part of the original email, but we also gave out the Most Improved Player Throphy. The winner really did improve over the course of the season.

Lineup and Playing Time:

I intend to rotate players liberally, though we will not put your kids at positions they cannot handle (like if you cannot catch, you will not play First Base).

These days kids pitch for their Travel Teams. Please email me with pitching conflicts.

Uniforms:

We will likely get our uniforms just before the first game.

Expect a 'get it to me right now' email from me on Team Snap very soon regarding numbers and uniform sizes (I know you already inputted this information, but ULLL likes to double-check).

Game Schedule:

The game schedule will be released in about a week.

Practices:

Our home field is Scott Jenkins 4 (SJ4), except after we 'Fall Back' practices will revert to there once a week

Until the games start (~about 3 weeks):

Tuesdays 5:30-7 at Haske

Thursdays 5-7 at SJ4

Saturdays 3-5 at Haske

Odds and Ends:

I expect all players to be at all team events. An email with conflicts, generally, travel takes priority over ULLL, and games take priority over practices.

Signs – We will use the second sign, and we will put our signs 'in' at the second practice... it is vitally important that your Player attend!

Coaching responsibilities:

Chris – Outfield

Jamie – Infield

Ryan – Hitting and Bunting

Kevin – Pitchers and Catchers

Always Rules:

1. Do your best; this way, you will not be faulted for lack of effort

2. Wear a cup, pants, and hat to practice and bring water, be prepared!

- Tuck shirt/jersey into pants

3. Run on the field (coaches walk), and run onto the field

- The 9/5 rule: We want all 9 of our guys, ready to field, in their defensive positions before 5 of their guys get off the field – every half inning

4. Respect your teammates, coaches, and the other team/coaches

5. Look at the ball and cover your bases!

Never Rules:

1. Cheat or lie – stealing is only allowed in baseball

2. Step on the lines; it is bad luck

3. Be last

4. Pick a ball up with your bare hand, unless it stops moving completely

5. Have your shirt/jersey untucked (the game will likely stop, and the Umpire will ask you to tuck it in), or look disheveled in any way

Thursday, August 13, 2021

1- Fields open next week, so our first practice is Tuesday, August 17 – 5:30 at Haske Field

2 - From Mario...There are currently no COVID-19 restrictions that have been placed on outdoor sports activities in Loudoun County. We are monitoring the situation, and if something changes, we will send out updates accordingly.

Monday, August 16, 2021

The first three weeks of practices have been added to Team Snap so you can mark your availability. Practice times will be adjusted once we get the game schedule. Please check your email/TeamSnap between 2:30 and 3:30 tomorrow in case we have to cancel due to the weather.

Tuesday, August 17, 2021

Today's practice plan is attached. Stay tuned for an update on field conditions. We will likely try to use the cages even if the field is closed. Please let me know through email or Team Snap if you will not be at practice.

Friday, August 20, 2021

Thanks for a great practice. Chris, and especially Ryan, are my heroes. Medical release form and trophy money to Kelly on Saturday, please. Thank you to those who have already turned these in.

Several players seemed confused by our signs, and one even asked for a hard copy of them (which I was happy to give). We will go over them again at practice, but here they are... please go over them with your players:

Signs are our secret – not to be shared with anyone!

Pitching

- Second sign from Coach Kevin to Catcher, who then signals the pitcher
- The difference between different pitches is in the grips
- Touch to brim of cap is 4 seam fastball (this is a slight change)
- Touch to nose is a curveball
- Touch to chin is change up
- A fourth sign is to touch the chest for a fourth pitch if the pitcher has one.
- All the rest are garbage meant to confuse the other team
- The Catcher then signals the Pitcher, 1, 2, 3, 4.

Hitting

- Before every pitch, look at the 3rd base coach when you are up
- Second sign from the 3rd Base Coach, step out of the box with your back foot before every pitch and let the 3rd Base Coach know you have got the sign by tapping your helmet
- Take (take the pitch, do not swing) – "L" with right arm
- Bunt – swipe across belt
- Hit – hit top of head

Baserunning

- Before every pitch, look at the 3rd Base Coach when you are on base
- We will run like we stole something – almost every pitch
- Big secondary leads, expect to run when you are on base
- Steal – swipe up and down pant leg.
- Jamie will be the Third Base Coach, with a backup of Ryan. Ryan will be the First Base Coach, with a backup of Chris.

Saturday, August 21, 2021

Good Morning,

Today's practice plan is attached. See everyone at 3:00, Haske Field.

Later in the Day…

Many thanks to all who helped. It was a great practice; I think the boys learned and had fun. I, for one, learned I should put directions on my rotations (which I will do - hey, we are all learning).

We still need trophy money from O and JM, and we have medical release forms from BR, JW, Bl, M, S, and W. In particular, ULLL takes the forms very seriously (I am just waiting for the email about them). Please get the needed forms and cash to Kelly at practice.

Practice next Tuesday, 5:30-7:00, at Haske. 1 2 3 get better.

Monday, August 23, 2021

Quote of the day:

"Baseball is like Church. Many attend but few understand." - Leo Durocher

This quote highlights the mental side of the game, which is very important. The boys should think of this when they hear Coach Ryan talk about "baseball IQ."

Scrimmage opportunity:

The Mighty Mussels have offered to scrimmage on Monday, August 30th, 5-7:15 at HE1. Please mark your availability in Team Snap. We will use this to replace our Tuesday practice that week if we have enough players.

Tuesday, August 24, 2021

Quote of the day:

"You can observe a lot by watching." - Yogi Berra

Remind the boys to pay attention during practice and during the games.

Yogi Berra is my favorite, and was a genius.

Today's practice plan is attached. See you at Haske 5:30-7.

Later in the Day...

Many thanks to Ryan, Chris, and Kelly for their help tonight. The practice would not have been possible without them. I think the kids learned and had fun.

Practice Thursday, Scott Jenkins 4, 5:00 to 7:30. This is a change of time; we will end 30 minutes early to avoid darkness. 1 2 3 get better.

Wednesday, August 25, 2021

Next Week

All,

Our scrimmage and practice schedule has cleared up for next week. I was only able to arrange 1 scrimmage, though I really tried hard for 2. As promised, we will only get together 3 times a week. Here's the deal:

Monday, August 30, 2021

We will scrimmage the Mighty Mussels at Hamilton Elementary 1, from 5:00 - 7:15, with 15 minutes of warmups (which should give us time to do about 1/2 of our normal pre-game routine). Please arrive at 4:50, ready to go. Alert me soon with any conflicts (within 24 hours of getting this message). If I do not hear anything from you, I will assume you are coming.

Players, please wear white or light tops, white or light pants. A River Bandits hat is preferred, or another dark hat if you do not have a River Bandits cap. The rest is up to you, though I would go with dark socks and belt. Coaches, I do not care.

There are some special rules for this scrimmage:

- A coach will call balls and strikes for our pitcher. It may be this way for real games, ULLL, apparently, does not have enough Umpires.

- Instead of 3 outs and swap, we will swap offense/defense after 30 pitches, and clear the bases at 3 outs.

- There will be 2 coaches on the field for defense to help players understand where to line up. For us, that will be Jamie and Chris.

- Remember, and remind players, we are always in bunt 1, and (even though we have not gone over this yet, coming to a practice soon) the Catcher will call 1st and 3rd defense. In both cases, the coaching staff will suggest changes to the players.

Tuesday, August 31, 2021

Practice is canceled, like I said, 3 times a week.

Wednesday 1 September

No practice or scrimmage

Thursday 2 September

Regular Practice at Scott Jenkins 4, 5:00-7:30. Please note the end time.

Friday 3 September

No practice or scrimmage

Saturday 4 September

Regular Practice at Haske 3:00 - 5:00

Games should start Labor Day week (6 September); everything will change. There is no game schedule yet. We will populate Team Snap with games as soon as we can. I will also send out the game schedule to you all. When they do start, expect 1 practice a week at Scott Jenkins 4. We may schedule rained-out games for our practice time.

There is no word on jerseys, though I would expect to have them and hats before our first game. I know they have been ordered, and as soon as I get them, you will get them. Expect an out-of-cycle get-together for that. More details to follow.

Please let me know if you have questions.

Thursday, August 26, 2021

All,

Attached is today's practice plan. See you at SJ4 at 5:00.

Saturday, August 28, 2021

Quote of the day:

"In the beginning, there was no baseball. But ever since, there have been few beginnings as good as the start of a new baseball season. It is the most splendid time in sport." - BJ Phillips (1981)

Today's practice plan is attached. See everyone at 3:00.

Sunday, August 29, 2021

Daily affirmation first:[15]

"The diamonds and the rituals of baseball create an elegant, trivial, enchanted grid on which our suffering shapeless sinful day leans for the momentary grace of order." -Donald Hall

"Baseball and the Meaning of Life" (1985)

Plan for the week:

Monday, 30 August 2021

We will scrimmage the Mighty Mussels at Hamilton Elementary 1, from 5:00 - 7:15. Please arrive at 4:50, ready to go. I only heard from one of you and will plan accordingly.

Players, please wear white or light tops, white or light pants. A River Bandits hat is preferred, or another dark hat if you do not have a River Bandits cap. The rest is up to you, though I would go with dark socks and belt. Coaches, wear whatever. Jamie will coach third, and Ryan will coach first. When we are on defense, two coaches, Jamie and Chris will be in the field. Jamie will call balls and strikes for us. There are some special rules for the scrimmage which I previously sent.

Game plan is attached...

Tuesday 31 August

Practice is canceled.

---

[15] I started calling the quotes affirmations.

Wednesday 1 September

No practice or scrimmage

Thursday 2 September

Regular Practice at Scott Jenkins 4, 5:00-7:00. Please note the end time. I was surprised by how it got dark so fast last week. I guess it gets late early - to preview a Berra quote.

Friday 3 September

No practice or scrimmage

Saturday, September 4, 2021

Regular Practice at Haske 3:00 - 5:00

Monday, August 30, 2021

Daily affirmation:

"It gets late early out there."

- Yogi Berra (referring to LF and the shadows at Yankee Stadium)

Scrimmage today, show time 4:50 at HE1.

Bonus… We lost the scrimmage

Well, that was interesting...

Quote of the Day:

"Whoever wants to know the heart and mind of America had better learn baseball."

-Jacques Barzun "God's country and mine" (1954)

Tuesday 31 August, 2021

This is just a reminder that practice is canceled today because of the scrimmage last night.

Since it looks like Thursday will be a rainout, maybe I should have held practice tonight? Nah, cannot time the weather; there is a quote about that (forthcoming).

Expect when we get together, there will be a healthy dose of remedial training (last night exposed some flaws).

Wednesday, September 1 2021

Daily Affirmation:

"Baseball is the only field of endeavor where a man can succeed three times out of ten and be considered a good performer." Ted Williams

In fact, if you get a hit 3/10, and do not use performance-enhancing drugs, you will make the Hall of Fame!

I have no idea whether the county will close SJ4 tomorrow, where we have practice 5-7. You will know as soon as I do, and I will make a practice plan.

Did you know you can configure the LCPS rainout line such that it will give you email (at about 2:30 each day) updates on specific fields? You only get an email when field status changes. Let me know if you need help.

Bonus, we were far from Little League World Series Quality.

Please see the following video from the LLWS:

https://www.littleleague.org/videos/recap-michigan-defeats-ohio-for-llbws/?utm_source=ll+-+august&utm_medium=email&utm_campaign=michigan+llbws-champs-video+link

Thursday, September 2, 2021

All,

First, our daily affirmation:

"Don't look back. Something might be gaining on you." - Satchel Paige

I have no idea if SJ4 will be open today, we have practice 5:00-7:00. It is closed right now. We will continue to monitor and let you know, a practice plan for today is attached.

This week's "immediate action required" was about volunteer forms - next week it will be about medical release forms. We still need medical release forms from O, JM, JH, and MH. We need trophy money ($10) from O and JM - please bring to Saturday's practice to be safe.

Yesterday I fielded (pun intended) a question about the game schedule. The game schedule has not been set (they seem to be waiting to schedule games with Central Loudoun Little League (CLLL)). We will get our uniforms (two shirts and a hat) before the first game. You should get them if you have not already: white pants, a black belt and socks.

Friday, September 3, 2021

First, our daily affirmation:

"I think Little League is wonderful. It keeps the kids out of the house." -Yogi Berra

Many thanks to Jamie for running practice last night.

The game schedule was released last night and is attached to this email. It is also on the ULLL website (ULLL.org). We will load it into team snap today.

Saturday, September 4, 2021

We got our uniforms and hats today at practice. If you got yours, please let me know if they do not fit.

If you were not at practice today, I have your uniforms and hats. If you must, and are in town, we are around this weekend and you can stop by our house and get yours - just around the corner from Haske. Otherwise, Kelly will have them at the next practice – September 7, 5:30 to 7:00 at Haske.

Sunday, September 5, 2021

First our daily affirmation:

"Age is a case of mind over matter. If you do not mind, it doesn't matter." -Satchel Paige

Plan of the week:

Tuesday 9/7, practice Haske 5:30-7:00

Wednesday 9/8, Game vs the Iron Birds at Mountain View ES at 5:30

Saturday 9/10, Game vs the Grizzlies at Haske 1 at 4:00 HOME

Remember: show time for games is 30 minutes prior, ready to go. So 5:00 and 3:30 this week.

Remember: when we are the Home Team (as we are next Saturday) we have to line the field, and I cannot do it. Chris has the primary responsibility, though he can assemble the masses to help. It would be good for this to be done prior to our 30-minute warmup.

I am canceling practice Thursday – we will only get together 3 times a week.

Tuesday will be our last practice at Haske owing to conflicts with other games. Effective Wednesday 9/8, I am canceling all practices at Haske. We will practice Thursdays at Scott Jenkins 4 from 4:30 until dark starting next week. Be on the lookout for specific times from me as we go, but I plan to start at 4:30 and go from there. I will say that if we do not have at least 60 minutes together, it is a bit of a waste, so look for me to cancel once we cannot practice until 5:30. Effectively, this means once we 'Fall Back', we will not practice anymore. I have asked about lighted fields, but it is unlikely we will get one because they are being used for games. I have done this in previous Fall seasons. Kelly will update the Team Snap calendar accordingly this weekend. Please note Kelly is a relative novice at all of this; take it easy on her while letting her know when things do not quite look right.

Attached, please find our game schedule in excel. I have found this very handy. Perhaps several of you are way ahead of me.

Monday, September 6, 2021

Our daily affirmation:

"A kid copies what is good. I remember the first time I saw Lefty O'Doul, and he was as far away as those palms. And I saw the guy come to bat in batting practice. I was looking through a knothole, and I said, 'Geez, does that guy look good!' And it was Lefty O'Doul, one of the greatest hitters ever." -Ted Williams

My better half suggested that 4:30 pm might be too early to start practice because the Middle Schoolers on the team might not be off the bus yet. Please let me know if you have a conflict and come late. This is really all about the light (and dark). There are not any lighted fields (I checked) for us to practice on.

And I did send a practice plan…

Tuesday 7 September, 2021

"All pitchers are liars or crybabies."

-Yogi Berra

Game plan for tomorrow attached.

And Uniforms…

We are green (away) jerseys tomorrow, but please bring both just in case we have a mix-up. I know this is the opposite of what Ryan and I said at practice. I just saw an email to managers from this morning that confirms yellow is home and green is away.

Wednesday, September 8, 2021

We have a game today. Show time is 5:00, as the team snap said - wear green today, bring yellow. Green is the road jersey, but you never know what the other team is going to do. I am tracking Greg, JH, and M will need to leave around 7 pm, and O will be late. Anything else?

"I think the baseball field must be the most beautiful thing in the world. It's so honest and precise. And we play on it. Every star gets humbled; every mediocre player has a great moment." -Lowell Cohn

"The Temple of Baseball" (1981)

Thursday, September 9, 2021

Practice is canceled tonight, and our next team event is a game at Haske, Saturday 4:00; show time is 3:30, ready to go regardless of what the schedule in team snap says. We are home against the Grizzlies; please wear yellow. Chris lines the field.

Daily Affirmation (I thought about "Babe Ruth is dead, throw strikes"):

"A nickel ain't worth a dime anymore." -Yogi Berra

Ah, the game last night. By my count, we lost 19-1 and were saved 3 times by the 5-run rule (in the Fall, any team may score a maximum of 5 runs in a half-inning). I think two things contributed to our huge loss.

First, the players on our team did not execute the fundamentals we talked about in practice. There were too many fundamental lapses to list. The little things add up, trust me. I will only say three things about this (I could say much more): they're in Majors now and are expected to know the fundamentals, so please study (this is the reason I send out practice plans). And your sons will not play for a travel team or the High School if they do not know them cold. And it gets late early; they are already being assessed. The good news is I have written them down for you. I am happy to send you a summary. The really good news is that we will keep practicing them and will keep working on them in games (it's a long season). Getting exposed at such a young age is a big advantage.

Second, we rotated inexperienced Pitchers (see all the walks, which are a killer), whereas the other team relied on 2 really good, experienced Pitchers and constrained their lineup. It would have been a different story if we Pitched S, JM, M, or C and went with a constrained lineup. I think we will see this over and over again. The good news is that I will stick with the rotational plan at least until everybody pitches. Fall is meant to be an instructional league, and it is important for the kids to gain experience. For what it is worth the old Kevin would have made the switch weeks ago and would have had practice tonight ;-). He would also be freaking out right now (I am not).

Friday, September 10, 2021

"All managers are losers; they are the most expendable pieces of furniture on the face of the Earth" -Ted Williams (and I beg to differ)

We have nothing today, show tomorrow is 3:30, ready to go.

Haske Rule: No gum or sunflower seeds. There are drains that get clogged easily. If River Bandits show at Haske with seeds or gum, I, or the coaches will make them throw it out.

An important rule, there were lots of these little things of which to keep track – It would have been challenging if I was whole.

Saturday, September 11, 2021 – A special day

We have a game today vs the Grizzlies. Show is 3:30, at Haske. Please wear yellow. Chris lines the field. A game plan is attached, please comment. There will be a moment of silence for 9/11* before the game. It is the least we can do. We get to play baseball on a beautiful Saturday because others have sacrificed. Let us never forget that.

Daily affirmation:

"After I got that hit off Satchel (Paige), I knew I was ready for the big leagues." -Joe DiMaggio

9/11 – It is important to teach the boys of our solemn responsibility on this day.

*Also, 11 September 2001 is very special to me. My Cousin, Alphonse Niedermeyer (google him), was one of the Port Authority Police Officers killed in the Twin Towers on that day. Al was a bona fide hero before 9/11. In fact, he was commended by the mayor (Dinkins) in 1993 for diving into the water when a US Airways flight skidded off the runway at LaGuardia. Al broke an arm and several ribs that day, but that did not matter to him. Human interest story - Al's wife Nancy had the last so-called 9/11 baby, early in March 2002 (Angelica Joy). Al never knew they were pregnant. In a twist of irony, Al's Father, Al, worked in security at the World Trade Center in 1993 when Terrorists bombed the WTC. He was in Security for a good long while (about 10 years), and I got tours (which I remember). My Cousin Al is the

reason I worked for the government. I decided to forego Academia in 2004 and apply my skills to the terrorist problem. I could say much more but will stop there.

Sunday, September 12, 2001

First, let's take care of a little business. We lost 14-8 yesterday. We played really well at the beginning (and for most of the game) and were ahead 8-6 after 5. I was very proud of the boys' effort; they clearly had been studying. Thank you. They should keep studying.

Since the boys seem really concerned with the score (score does not count in the Fall), please tell them I am keeping it in the dirt outside the dugout. I learned a couple of lessons yesterday that will stick with me. First, save a pitcher for the 6th. I assumed we would not play the 6th (bad assumption). Second, it is all about Pitching and Catching. They scored 8 runs in that last inning because we could not throw it over the plate and could not catch it. Expect a somewhat constrained lineup, particularly at Pitcher and Catcher, when we next get together.

Daily Affirmation:

"90 feet between the bases is the nearest thing to perfection that Man has yet achieved." -Red Smith, Broadcaster, (1908-1982).

BTW No truer words have ever been spoken. At 90 feet (We play at 60), a crisply hit ball to SS will result in an out by a step, if the batter is running hard. Score that 6-3 if you are keeping score at home.

Plan for the week:

*Please note that show time for all games is actually 1 hour prior to the game. Kelly will adjust (er, readjust) the Team Snap. In the meantime, please continue to rely on these emails.

Weds (9/15), we are at Freedom Park in Leesburg, on Huber field. Show is 5:30, Game (vs the CLLL White Sox) is at 6:30. We are the road team, which means we will wear green, occupy the 3rd base dugout, and take the field for warmups immediately for 25 minutes, then we hit.

Thurs (9/16), we have practice at SJ4 4:30-6:30

Saturday (9/18), we are at Haske. Show is 3:00, Game (vs the ULLL Iron Pigs) is at 4:00. We are the home team, which means we will wear yellow, occupy the 1st base dugout, and hit 1 hour before the game, and take the field after.

The local rules for pre-game warm-ups are attached.

Monday, September 13, 2021

Baseball is ninety percent mental. The other half is physical." - Yogi Berra

Study, study, study…

Tuesday, September 14, 2021

First, let's do our daily affirmation:

"A man has to have goals - for a day, for a lifetime - and that was mine, to have people say, 'There goes Ted Williams, the greatest hitter who ever lived.'" -Ted Williams

Tomorrow we have a game in Leesburg at 6:30, show is 5:30. Let me know if you cannot make it. I will be a little scarce today, but I will get back to you. A game plan for tomorrow is attached; you are invited to comment.

Wednesday, September 15, 2021

First:

"Ain't no man can avoid being born average, but there ain't no man got to be common." -Satchel Paige

We have a game today in Leesburg (Freedom Park - Huber). Show is at 5:30. I did not hear from any of you, so I think everyone can make it.

Matty may not play (we are waiting on a COVID test); such is life in 2021. He is fine; we think it's just allergies.

I will be scares again today, but let me know if you have questions, and I will get back to you.

Thursday, September 16, 2021

Though we lost 5-2 last night, the boys played, hands down, their best game. After seeing the other team warm-up I was worried we would lose 20 or 25 to nothing. The boys are really learning and growing. Keep Studying! Your efforts are appreciated.

We have practice today 4:30-6:30 at Scott Jenkins 4. I am tracking no S or M, and that W may be late. What else? I will send a practice plan later (I am shooting for 1200, and I have one in draft) and let you know if the field is actually open (we got a lot of rain last night) around 2:30.

Daily Affirmation:

"Any baseball is beautiful. No other small package comes as close to the ideal in design and utility. It is a perfect object for a man-made pick-it-up, and it instantly suggests its purpose. It is meant to be thrown a considerable distance thrown hard and with precision." -Roger Angell, Five Seasons (1977)

Friday, September 17, 2021

We have nothing today. Daily affirmation:

"Bill Dickey is learning me his experience." -Yogi Berra

Bill Dickey and Yogi Berra are the only players from a major sports franchise to have the same number retired. In this, special, case 8 is retired twice by the Yankees.

Saturday, September 18, 2021

We have a game today at Haske vs. the ULLL Iron Pigs. The game is at 4:00, show is at 3:00. We are the home team, please wear yellow. Greg lines the field. A game plan is attached. I am tracking no S or Chris. Any others?

Daily Affirmation:

"Baseball gives every American boy a chance to excel, not just to be as good as someone else but to be better than someone else. This is the nature of man and the name of the game." Ted Williams

Sunday, September 19, 2021

We lost last night's game. Suffice it to say, the boys need to pay attention to the coaches and their fundamentals. I could say much more. We should have won. We picked up two bottles and (I think) a Fitbit (I did have it in my hand). We will be around this afternoon before about five pm if you would like to pick them up; we live right around the corner from Haske. Otherwise, we will bring them to the game on Wednesday.

Plan for the week:

Wednesday (9/22), Game Hamilton Elementary 1, 5:30 (4:30 show), we are the visitor, wear green.

Thursday (9/23), Practice, Scott Jenkins 4, 4:30-6:30

Saturday (9/25), Game, Haske, 4:00 (3:00 show), we are home, wear yellow

"He (Bill Veeck) asked me to throw at a cigarette as a plate and I threw four out of five over it." A far cry from us. -Satchel Paige

Monday, September 20, 2021

"He hits from both sides of the plate. He's amphibious." -Yogi Berra

Tuesday, September 21, 2021

Today is Tuesday, and we have nothing today. A game plan for tomorrow is attached, please comment.

Daily Affirmation:

"Man may penetrate the outer reaches of the universe. He may solve the very secret of eternity itself. But for me, the ultimate human experience is to witness the flawless execution of the hit and run." -Branch Rickey (Dodgers General Manager 1943-1950)

Wednesday, September 22, 2021

We have a game today vs. the Tides. Show time is 4:30 at Hamilton Elementary for a 5:30 game. Please wear green. We are the road team and will occupy the third base dugout.

If we get rained out, we will try to reschedule for one of our practice times.

I will be in touch.

A practice plan for tomorrow is attached. Please comment, and I reserve the right to change it, particularly if we play a game.

Daily Affirmation:

"How can you hit and think at the same time?"

-Yogi Berra

It rained, and we did not play. Tragic.

Thursday, September 23, 2021

I will take the mystery out of it - practice today is canceled! Enjoy your time off. SJ4 is currently closed, and if it opens (the rain will stop, and the sun may come out), it is likely to be too wet.

This means we may not practice again. Next week we have three games, the week after that we 'Fall Back.' I will consult with the coaches and see if we want to break my rule and get together 4 times next week and practice on 9/30. More to follow...

Daily Affirmation:

"Baseball's future? Bigger and bigger, better and better! No question about it, it's the greatest game there is!" Amen. -Ted Williams

Friday, September 24, 2021

Today is Friday, and we do not have anything today.

Daily Affirmation:

"The clock doesn't matter in baseball. Time stands still or moves backward. Theoretically, one game could go on forever. Some seem to." -Herb Caen, San Francisco Chronicle (1978)

Saturday, September 25, 2021

We have a game today. Wear yellow. Show is 3 pm at Haske for a 4 pm game vs. the Emeralds.

We are the home team. Greg lines the field. Game plan is attached. I am tracking no Chris or S. Anyone else?

Oh, we will practice on Thursday, 9/30, and get together 4 times this week.

"How old would you be if you did not know how old you were?" -Satchel Paige

Sunday, September 26, 2021

We lost 14-2 in the game yesterday. I could say lots, but I will only say here that the boys need to be baseball ready on every play - like the Emeralds were. They made a number of great plays. That's life, is it not? The line drives get caught, and the bloopers fall in.

Plan for the week:

We get together 4 times!

Monday 9/27 - Game at SJ1, wear green, show 5:00, game 5:30. This is a rescheduled game due to rain, note show time. There will be a shortened warm-up period. We will definitely do the throwing program and run a pole. A game plan is attached, please comment.

Wednesday 9/29, Game Freedom-Reavis (Leesburg), wear green, 5:30 show, 6:00 game

Thursday 9/30, practice SJ4, 4:30 - 6:30

Friday, 10/1, Game vs. CLLL Giants, wear yellow (we are home), 5:30 show for a 6:30 game, Chris lines the field

Daily Affirmation:

"I always thought that record would stand until it was broken." -Yogi Berra

Monday, September 27, 2021

We have a game against the Tides today at SJ1. Wear green, show is 5:00 for a 5:30 game. This is a makeup for a rainout, and there will be a shortened warm-up period. I want the boys to do the throwing program and run a pole before the game.

Daily affirmation:

"By the time you know what to do, you're too old to do it."
How true. -Ted Williams

Tuesday, September 28, 2021

First, "I believe in the Rip Van Winkle theory - That a man
from 1910 must be able to wake up after being asleep for 70 years,
walk into a baseball park and understand baseball perfectly." -
Bowie Kuhn (Baseball Commissioner 1969-84)

Second, we have a game tomorrow in Leesburg @ Freedom-
Reavis 6:30 game, 5:30 show. Wear green again. A game plan is
attached, please comment.

Third, we lost 14-7 in the darkness shortened game yesterday.
My better half (who's always right) told me to say we made a lot of
great plays, and we will see you Wednesday. I will add, because I
cannot help myself, that the boys need to be baseball ready on
every pitch and field with the two hands God gave them.

Wednesday, September 29, 2021

First, our daily affirmation:

"I ain't ever had a job; I just always played baseball." -Satchel
Paige

We have a game today. 5:30 show in Leesburg @ Freedom
Park Reavis Field. Please wear green. I did not hear from anyone,
so I assume everyone can make it.

We have practice tomorrow, 4:30-6:30 at SJ4. A practice plan
is attached. Please comment. And, I reserve the right to change it.

For future planning - there is a game on Friday at Haske with a 5:30 show, and we will wear yellow.

Thursday, September 30, 2021

We have practice today at SJ4 4:30-6:30. I am tracking that W will be late, and S and M will not be there. Any others?

We have a game tomorrow at Haske against the CLLL Giants. Showtime is 5:30. Wear yellow; we are the home team. Chris lines the field.

I intend to send the game plan for tomorrow by noon today.

Daily Affirmation:

"(Joe) DiMaggio was the greatest all-around player I ever saw. His career cannot be summed up in numbers and awards. It might sound corny, but he had a profound and lasting impact on the country." -Ted Williams, who played with Joe's brother Dom

About last night... We lost 13-7 (the scoreboard was wrong), but it was much closer than that. I was heartened to see JH pitch much better in his 2nd inning, and a number of other good things happened (including us having the lead late).

Friday, October 1, 2021

First, "Baseball is the only thing besides the paperclip that hasn't changed."

-Bill Veeck, Indians Owner 1946-1950

We have a game tonight. The game is at Haske, and show time is 5:30. Please wear yellow. We are the home team, and Chris lines the field. An updated game plan is attached - remember we only have 8.

Saturday, October 2, 2021

The boys fought valiantly last night, with only 8 players. A number of the kids got to play positions they have not played in a while or before, and I was proud of them. Monday, we have a game against the Mighty Mussels (Haske, we are the home team, please wear yellow, 5:30 show for a 6:30 game, Chris lines the field) and I would really like us to play well. Please remember (and remind the boys) to be baseball ready on every pitch and field with two hands, and I would add, when hitting, stand close to the plate.* And, be ready; I am thinking of having practice Thursday, I will make a final determination tomorrow, please comment.

Daily Affirmation:

"I can see how he (Sandy Koufax) won twenty-five games. What I do not understand is how he lost five." -Yogi Berra

Let me know if you have questions.

-Coach Kevin

* I think ball fear is an issue for some on the team. I was cured of ball fear when I was about 10 when my Little League (LL) Coach lined us all up behind home plate and lined a bucket of balls at us from between the plate and the pitcher's mound. We either caught the balls or, well, got hit. That would never fly now. What I will say is that if you get hit while batting, I have a standing rule that you steal second on the next pitch, so you get a double. And, it only hurts for a second.

Sunday, October 3, 2021

First, "I don't generally like running. I believe in training by rising gently up and down from the bench." -Satchel Paige

Second, a plan for the week:

Monday, 4th October, Game vs. Mighty Mussels, show 5:30 for a 6:30 game. Haske, wear yellow - we are home; Chris lines the field. We are on the first base side. A game plan is attached, please comment, and remember, I would really like to play well.

Thursday 7 October, practice SJ4, 4:30-6:30; I am tracking W will be late and no S. What else?

Saturday 9 October, Game vs. The Trash Pandas, show 3:00 for a 4:00 game. Mountain View ES, wear green; we are the road team and will occupy the third-base side.

Monday, October 4, 2021

First, "Hitting is fifty percent above the shoulders." - Ted Williams

Second, we have a game today. 5:30 show at Haske vs. The Mighty Mussels, wear yellow (we are home and will be on the first base side), Chris lines the field, and I really want to play well, so make extra sure the boys are ready. A game plan is attached.

Tuesday, October 5, 2021

First, "No game in the world is as tidy and dramatically neat as baseball. With cause and effect, crime and punishment, motive and result, so cleanly defined." -Paul Gallico (1897-1976) sportswriter

Second, we have practice Thursday, 4:30-6:30 at SJ4. I am tracking that W will be late, no M, and S is TBD (has his situation for Thursday cleared up?). Anybody else?

Third, we lost again last night 10-5, but we could have won, and the boys played, I thought their best game of the season. They have really improved. There were several highlights, including S, who was a terror on the bases (and was safe at home, btw), W got a big hit, and M really played well.

Finally, we have a game on Saturday at Mountain View Elementary School (MVES) against the Trash Pandas. If we play as well as we played last night, we will win. Show is 3:00pm. Please wear green. We are the road team and will occupy the 3rd base dugout. I am tracking no S (or Chris) and no BR. Anyone else (my better half tells me no C also). We can play with 8, but less than that, we will have to forfeit, although the game might get rained out.

Wednesday, October 6, 2021

First, we do not have anything today. We do have practice tomorrow, SJ4 4:30-6:30. I am tracking that W will be late, and we will be missing C, M, and S. No Timmy, or Aaron, but the other Coaches should be there. Anyone else? A practice plan is attached. You should also know that I offered up Thursday, 10/14 to make up for this Saturday if we get rained out (rain is in the forecast), so we might get together next Thursday. More to follow.

Second, daily affirmation:

"It's like deja vu all over again." -Yogi Berra

Thursday, October 7, 2021

We have practice today 4:30-6:30 at SJ4. I am tracking that W will be late, and S, M, and C will not be there. Any others? We will let you know if the field is closed.

Daily Affirmation:

"I don't know what you're going to do, Mr. (Dizzy) Dean, but I'm not going to give up any runs if we have to stay here all night." -Satchel Paige

Friday, October 8, 2021

Frist, "Baseball to me is still the national pastime because it is a summer game. I feel that most Americans are summer people. That Summer is what they think of when they think of their childhood. I think it stirs up an incredible emotion within people." -Steve Busby, Royals Pitcher (1972-80)

We have a game tomorrow; game plan is attached. We have only 8 and it might rain. If we do get rained out, the Manager of the Trash Pandas and I are discussing playing on Tuesday or Thursday, more to follow. I will try for Thursday. Anyway, for tomorrow, we are the road team, wear green, we will occupy the 3rd base dugout, and show time is 3:00 for a 4:00 game at MVES.

Saturday, October 9, 2021

First, we will play today. It looks like the rain will hold off. As a reminder, we only have 8; a game plan is attached. It is a 3 pm show for a 4 pm game at Mountain View Elementary School. Please wear green, and we will occupy the 3rd Base Dugout.

Second, "Hitting is the most important part of the game. It is where big money is, where much of the status is, and the fan interest." - Ted Williams

Sucks, there were a lot of changes to the schedule. The weather was a constant worry, though it was not the issue this time.

Later…Sorry for the multiple messages, but I only *just* heard back from the opposing Manager. Today's game will be played at 5 pm on Thursday.

Sunday, October 10, 2021

All, first, "If a man can beat you, walk him." - Satchel Paige

Plan for the Week: 3 games, no practices (plan on not practicing again, though I will be in touch if we do decide to practice. Likely, we will need our practice time for make-up games, like this week).

Tuesday, 10/12, Game at Haske against the Grasshoppers. 5:30 show for a 6:30 game. Wear yellow - we are home and will be on the 1st base side. Chris lines the field.

Thursday, 10/14 Game at SJ4 against the Trash Pandas (this is the re-scheduled rainout from yesterday). We are away, wear green, and will occupy the 3rd base dugout. 4:00 show for a 5:00 game. Show if you can, and let me know if you will not be there by game time. 3 against the Iron Pigs. We are away, wear green, and will occupy the 3rd base dugout. 3:00 show for a 4:00 game.

Monday, October 11, 2021

We have a game tomorrow against The Grasshoppers. Please wear yellow, we are home and will occupy the 1st base side at Haske. 5:30pm show for a 6:30pm game. Chris lines the field. A game plan is attached, please comment.

Trophies are ordered.

Daily Affirmation:

"Boys would be Big Leaguers as everybody knows. But so would Big Leaguers be boys." -Philip Roth (The Great American Novel, 1973)

Tuesday, October 12, 2021

We have a game today against The Grasshoppers. Please wear yellow; we are home and will occupy the 1st base side at Haske. 5:30 pm show for a 6:30 pm game. Chris lines the field.

Daily Affirmation:

"I don't know (if they were men or women fans running naked across the field). They had bags over their heads." -Yogi Berra

Wednesday, October 13, 2021

About last night, we did not win - we tied (11-11). That said, let the boys keep thinking we won. They deserve it.

We have a makeup game tomorrow against the Trash Pandas. We are the road team - wear green, and we will occupy the 3rd base side at SJ4. Show is 4pm for a 5pm game. I am tracking no

Greg, no MH or BR and C (5:45) will be late. What else? A game plan is attached, please comment.

Daily Affirmation:

"If I was being paid thirty-thousand dollars a year, the very least I could do was hit .400" - Ted Williams Inflation.

Thursday, October 14, 2021

First, Daily Affirmation:

"I never rush myself. See, they can't start the game without me." -Satchel Paige

Second, we have a make-up game today at SJ4, show is 4:00. Wear green. I am tracking no BR or Greg, and W will be late (4:45/4:50), and C will be late (5:45). What else? An updated game plan is attached.

Third, IMPORTANT, our final game has been moved by Loudoun County Parks and Recreation (LCPR) to Friday 29 October at 6:00, 5:00 show. At this point, I do not know what it means for our end-of-season party and trophy celebration except that it will not be on 30 Oct.

The trophies have arrived. They look great!

Friday, October 15, 2021

Frist, Daily Affirmation:

"Growing up is a ritual - more deadly than religion, more complicated than baseball. For there seemed to be no rules. Everything was experienced for the first time. But baseball can soothe even those pains. For it is stable and permanent steady as a grandpa dozing on a wicker chair on the veranda." -W.P. Kinsella Shoeless Joe (1982)

Second, thanks to Jamie for Umpiring last night, and to the coaches for helping. We lost 10-4 if you were not keeping score.

Third, two important schedule items:

1. Our game on Saturday against the Iron Pigs might get rained out. If it does, we might play next Thursday (10/21). I am currently in discussions with the opposing Manager. It would be sort of like last night. A game plan is attached, please comment. I expect everyone but Greg.

2. We will do our party and trophy presentation Thursday, 10/28 5:30-6:30 at SJ4. Expect a sign-up genius soon.

Saturday, October 16, 2021

First, Daily Affirmation (one of my favorites of all time) "If people don't want to come out to the ballpark, how are you going to stop them?" -Yogi Berra

Second, we might have a game today; maybe not - we will see. If we get rained out, we still might play on the 21st. I will also be working with ULLL to reschedule on a lighted field (there are 2); more to follow. I will be in touch - via team snap. Show is 3:00, for a 4:00 game at Franklin Park 3. We are the road team. Please wear green. We will occupy the 3rd base dugout. I am tracking no BR or Greg. A game plan is attached. Please comment.

We play the Mudcats at Haske on Tuesday. We are home, please wear yellow, and will occupy the first base dugout. 5:30 show for a 6:30 game. Chris lines the field (for the last time). I am tracking no BR, anyone else? A game plan is attached. Please Comment.

Sunday, October 17, 2021

First, Daily Affirmation ~ "If there was ever a man born to be a hitter, it was me." - A modest Ted Williams

Second, I do not know yet about re-scheduling our rainout, it may be this Thursday (10/21), or it may not happen. I am working hard to get a favorable outcome for us. I will be in touch with an email.

Third, I do know: - Tuesday, 19 October, we play the Mudcats at Haske and are the home team. 5:30 show for a 6:30 game. We will occupy the 1st base dugout. Please wear yellow. Chris lines the field.

-Saturday, 23rd October, we play the Emeralds at Franklin Park 3. We are the road team, please wear green. 3:00 show for a 4:00 game.

Monday, October 18, 2021

First, a game plan for tomorrow is attached; we pay the Mudcats at Haske, 5:30 show for a 6:30 game. We are home, please wear yellow, and we will occupy the 1st base dugout. Chris lines the field.

Second, Daily Affirmation: "I never threw an illegal pitch. The trouble is, once in a while, I toss one that ain't never been seen by this generation." – Satchel Paige

Tuesday, October 19, 2021

First, Daily Affirmation, "I feel an invisible bond between the generations. An anchor of loyalty linking my sons to the grandfather whose face they never saw but whose person they have already come to know through the most timeless of all sports baseball." - Doris Kearns Godwin "From Father with Love" (1987)

Second, we have a game today vs the Mudcats at Haske. 5:30 show for a 6:30 game. We are home, please wear yellow, and we will occupy the 1st base dugout. Chris lines the field. I am tracking no BR or Greg - who else?

Third, A slight schedule change that doesn't affect our game times but does affect our opponents - Late breaking news - CLLL is unable to play the Majors games scheduled on 10/27. As a result, we have reworked the master schedule so the impacted ULLL teams will play one another instead. Here is the updated matchup:

Iron Birds vs. River Bandits at FP3 @ 6PM

Wednesday, October 20, 2021

First, "I'm a lucky guy, and I'm happy to be with the Yankees. And I want to thank everyone for making this night necessary." - Yogi Berra

Second, we have a game on 23 October at Franklin Park 3, against the Emeralds. We are the visitor, please wear green, and we will occupy the third-base dugout. Show time is 3:00 for a 4:00 game. A game plan is attached, please comment. Right now, we only have 8, and if we lose one more, we will have to forfeit. I am tracking no BR, O, JM, Jamie, Greg, and Ryan. Any others?

Third, there is no practice or game on 10/21. I tried.

Bet you thought you would go a day without an email from me. Never! Sorry I am late.

Thursday, October 21, 2021

First, "I hope somebody hits .400 soon. Then people can start pestering that guy with questions about the last guy to hit .400." - Ted Williams (the last person to hit .400 in MLB 1941, in case you did not know - there is a good story about that, suffice it to say that Ted Williams was a beast. Let me know if you would like the story).

Second, we do not have anything today; next is our game on Saturday.

Third, remember 'practice' next week, October 28, 5:30-6:30 at SJ4, is our pizza party and trophy presentation. Expect a sign-up genius for plates, drinks, cups, and the like today.

Fourth, both our games for next week have changed, the opponent for the 27th and the game on the 30th was moved to the 29th. We cannot change the game schedule in Team Snap (ULLL owns that). A useful view is attached.

Fifth, I bet you missed morning emails from me yesterday. We had computer issues and are getting a new one.

Let me know if you have questions.

Friday, October 22, 2021

First, "It's funny what a few no-hitters do for a body." – Satchel Paige.

Second, we have a game tomorrow vs the Emeralds; we have 8 players and are missing several coaches. Aaron will help. A game plan is attached, please let me know if you will not be there if you have not. We are the Visitor at Franklin Park. This is the best of all possible worlds in terms of things to do – we do not have to do anything. Please wear green and show at 3 pm for a 4 pm game. We will occupy the 3rd base dugout.

Third, remember 'practice' next week, October 28, 5:30-6:30 at SJ4, is our pizza party and trophy presentation. The sign-up genius is out, please sign up.

Saturday, October 23, 2021

First, "There have been only two geniuses in the world. Willie Mays and Willie Shakespeare." – Tallulah Bankhead (1903-1968, Actress)

Second, we have a game today vs the Emeralds at 4 pm at Franklin Park. We have 8 players and are missing several coaches. Aaron will help out. We are the Visitor. Please wear green and show at 3 pm. We will occupy the 3rd base dugout.

Third, 'practice' next week, October 28, 5:30-6:30 at SJ4, is our pizza party and trophy presentation. The sign-up genius is out, please sign up.

Bonus!

All, this is a good one: "When I was a small boy in Kansas, a friend of mine and I went fishing...I told him I wanted to be a real Major League Baseball Player. A genuine professional like Honus Wagner. My friend said he'd like to be President of the United

States. Neither of us got our wish." - Dwight D. Eisenhower (1890-1969, 34th President of the United States)

Sunday, October 24, 2021

First, "You gotta be a man to play baseball for a living. But you gotta have a lot of little boy in you." - Roy Campanella (Dodgers Catcher 1948-1957)

Second, thanks to Aaron for helping yesterday. Chris is rock solid. Though we were shorthanded, several new firsts made the game worthwhile.

Plan for the Week:

* please note both of our games for next week have changed.*

Wednesday, 27th October, Game against the Iron Birds at Franklin Park 3. 5 pm show for a 6:00 game. We are home, please wear yellow, and we will occupy the first base dugout.

Thursday 28 October, 'practice' 5:30-6:30 at Scott Jenkins 4, pizza party, and trophy presentation. The sign-up genius is out, please sign up. Rain date is 30 October at my house - just around the corner from Haske.

Friday, October 29, game vs the Mudcats at Franklin Park 3. 3 pm show for a 4 pm game. We are the road team. Please wear green, and we will occupy the third-base dugout.

Then the season is over.

Monday, October 25, 2021

First, "The strongest thing baseball has going for it today is its yesterdays. - Lawrence Ritter (The Glory of their Times, 1966).

Second, we have a game on Wednesday - Oct. 27th at Franklin Park 3 (FP3) against the Iron Birds. 5:00 pm show for a 6:00 pm game. We are home; please wear yellow, and I am expecting everyone except BR. Let me know if you cannot come; a game plan is attached, please comment.

First, "I've found that you don't need to wear a necktie if you can hit." - Ted Williams Amen, I wear a necktie.

Second, we actually won last night 16-12. It was good the boys got a win; it is good to see everyone is hitting now. Thanks to Jamie for Umpiring the whole game and then some, and the coaches, without whom this season would not have happened.

Third, our next and final game is still up in the air. I know it will be at Haske 6:00 game, 5:00 show. I know we will be the visitor, wear green, and occupy the 3rd base dugout. I know the game will not be tomorrow (rain) or 1 November (I, and many of you, need to go to Church). It will likely be on 2 or 3 November. Can you all play? What about BR? A game plan, such as it is, is attached. Please comment.

Finally, our party is tonight 5:30-6:30 at SJ4. Thank you to all who have signed up to bring stuff. We will have pizza and present trophies.

Saturday, October 30, 2021

First, there is no confirmation, but I think we will play 3 November with 100% certainty. I did not hear from anyone, so expect everyone. Jamie - you might have to umpire some more (like when we are pitching. Ha, you thought you were done!) Once confirmed, it will be at Haske 6:00 game, 5:00 show. I know we will be the visitor, wear green, and occupy the 3rd base dugout. I will let you know when we are confirmed.

Second, "The great thing about baseball is that there's a crisis every day." - Gabe Paul (Yankees General Manager, 1973-77).

Tuesday, November 2, 2021

First, "I've said it once, and I'll say it a hundred times, I'm forty-four years old." -Satchel Paige (me too)

Second, we have a game tomorrow - our last time together. I am tracking no O, anyone else? We will be at Haske 6:00 game, 5:00 show. We will be the visitor, wear green, and occupy the 3rd base dugout. Jamie may have to umpire.

Wednesday, November 3, 2021

We drove by Haske this morning, and the field was still a mess. We are also down to 7 players for tonight, so we are going to cancel. (November is not really baseball weather anyway).

Thank you for a great season! This was the last fall little league season for the Sweeney family and our fourth or fifth as River Bandits. It was a memorable one with a great group of players and coaches. Thank you for being so supportive and flexible. Enjoy your winter break, and I hope to see you all again in the spring.

Conclusion

I will conclude by just saying two things. First, it was an absolute honor to coach Matty's Little League team in the Fall, and it was critical to my recovery. I thank Mario (the former Vice President) and Kerry (the President) of Upper Loudoun Little League (ULLL) for giving me the opportunity. Second, I will say that season represented a major change in my coaching style and philosophy. I went from, before strokes, a Type A coach who only wanted to win games (and saw player development as a means to the end of winning) to a coach who genuinely cared about player development. I hope this comes through in my emails to the team. If it does not, there is this fact: We won once and tied once and lost the rest of our games, and I really did not care. I wanted the players to learn and have fun. They did, so I was successful.

I included a sample practice plan (I had 10s of these), along with a sample game plan (I had one of these for every game), and our game schedule from later in the season:

Fall 2021 Majors River Bandits – Sample Practice Plan

Thursday 16 September 2021

Scott Jenkins 4, 4:30-6:30

W will be late, No S or M, No T, A

4:30 Team Stretch and pole

4:40 Throwing Program

4:55 Water Break

Go over signs and bunt defenses

Go over that the 2B must back up the throw from C to P on every pitch

5:10 Follow your Throws Drill

1 Player at each base, the rest in a line at SS

Chris hits (or throws) ground balls to SS

SS throws to 1st, 1st throws to 2nd, 2nd throws to 3rd, 3rd throws to home. C goes to the end of the line at SS

1st, 2nd, 3rd, home must all do two-handed sweep tags

Players 'follow their throws' to the next base, C and 3rd base run in foul territory along the 3rd baseline

The other adult coaches direct traffic.

5:35 Water Break

Go over cut and cover (all situations, especially runners on 1st or 1st and 3rd and runner on 2nd, cover 2B, SS, P, and 1B responsibilities.)

Go over C responsibilities

The most important defensive position – Coach on the field

Before every pitch:

Get the pitch sign from Coach Kevin and signal the P

Call 3-digit 1st and 3rd play in front of the plate (go over plays 1, 2, 3, 4)

Make sure everyone is baseball ready

- Block everything. Always go to your knees and chest down – keep the ball in front of you. Explain the Mighty Ducks drill. They do not call Catcher's gear the tools of ignorance for nothing; you will get hit with the ball in the chest (hopefully!) where you have padding.
- It's called baseball because the object of the game is to accrue bases while keeping the other team from doing so. The Catcher is vitally important in this. The #1 way runs score in LL is via the passed ball.
- Helmet off (just toss it aside) to throw and catch fly balls.
- Pop time, or how fast you throw to bases, is the most important stat that college coaches look at.

5:45-6:30 Go over Pre- Game Routine

Do the full Monty (throwing program, IF/OF, and hitting)

Ryan hits, adult Coaches direct traffic

For hitting: Ryan pitches, Chris does the tee, Jamie, and Greg coach them up. I will help.

6:30 practice Ends

Ryan takes the team out

We do not have to do anything to SJ4

A sample game plan:

Batting Order	First Name	shirt #	1st	2nd	3rd	4th	5th	6th
1	M	16	C	C	RCF	P	RCF	LCF
2	S	28	P	RCF	2B	3B	LCF	1B
3	JA	5	SS	LCF	3B	LCF	2B	SS
4	W	3	2B	SS	1B	SS	C	3B
5	BR	15	RCF	2B	LCF	1B	SS	2B
6	C	1	1B	P	P	2B	3B	C
7	BL	2	3B	3B	SS	RCF	P	P
8	JO	27	LCF	1B	C	C	1B	RCF
Friday, 10/1 vs. CLLL-Giants, Haske, 6:30 game, 5:30 show								
No Greg								
No O or MH								
JO cannot pitch								

Figure 5: A Game Lineup

Our game schedule:

Date	Division	Home	Visitor	Field	Time	game #	liner/raker	lineup?
Wed, 09/08/2021	Majors (Fall)	IronBirds	River Bandits	MV	5:30 PM	1	N/A	Y
Sat, 09/11/2021	Majors (Fall)	River Bandits	Grizzlies	Haske 1	4:00 PM	2	Chris	Y
Wed, 09/15/2021	Majors (Fall)	CLLL-White Sox	River Bandits	Freedom-Huber	6:30 PM	3	N/A	Y
Sat, 09/18/2021	Majors (Fall)	River Bandits	IronPigs	Haske 1	4:00 PM	4	Greg	Y
Wed, 09/22/2021	Majors (Fall)	Tides	River Bandits	HE 1	5:30 PM	5	N/A	Y
Sat, 09/25/2021	Majors (Fall)	River Bandits	Emeralds	Haske 1	4:00 PM	6	Greg	Y
Wed, 09/29/2021	Majors (Fall)	CLLL-Phillies	River Bandits	Freedom-Reavis	6:30 PM	7	N/A	Y
Fri, 10/01/2021	Majors (Fall)	River Bandits	CLLL-Giants	Haske 1	6:30 PM	8	Chris	Y
Mon, 10/04/2021	Majors (Fall)	River Bandits	Mighty Mussels	Haske 1	6:30 PM	9	Chris	Y
Sat, 10/09/2021	Majors (Fall)	Trash Pandas	River Bandits	MV	4:00 PM	10	N/A	Y
Tue, 10/12/2021	Majors (Fall)	River Bandits	Grasshoppers	Haske 1	6:30 PM	11	Chris	Y
Sat, 10/16/2021	Majors (Fall)	IronPigs		FP 3	4:00 PM	12	N/A	Y
Tue, 10/19/2021	Majors (Fall)	River Bandits	Mudcats	Haske 1	6:30 PM	13	Chris	Y
Sat, 10/23/2021	Majors (Fall)	Emeralds	River Bandits	FP 3	4:00 PM	14	N/A	Y
Wed, 10/27/2021	Majors (Fall)	River Bandits	Iron Birds	FP 3	6:00 PM	15	N/A	Y
Wed, 11/03/2021	Majors (Fall)	Mudcats	River Bandits	Haske 1	6:00 PM	16	N/A	Y

Figure 6: Our Game Schedule

Chapter 5
The Land of Falling Trees

As I mentioned at the outset, this chapter will be about some of my more significant accomplishments since the strokes, which have much more to do with my physical progress than my inability to talk. I put these here so stroke recovery patients (and their families) may know what to expect. I have had some other accomplishments, which fall just short of being significant, and we will start there. Then I will go, chronologically, through my most significant accomplishments – that are summarized in Figure 7. My significant accomplishments tend to cluster at the end of 2021 and early 2022, with one notable exception. I do not know if there is a medical reason for this; for example, 'we would expect in 12-18 months Kevin will'… Going forward, I am sure I will have more firsts but intend to focus on getting faster – which I think will come (mostly) as I learn new, more efficient ways to do things (not necessarily, from my improvement, per se).

I had many accomplishments that fall short of significant, dating back to September 2020. There was a first time for everything, but I would highlight four events: getting my first COVID shot (at work), going back to work, the 'welcome back' party work had for me, and the physical progress that led me to walk for the first time. One thing is certain if I can do it, anybody, and you can. I had very serious strokes (Chapter 1) and was a middling athlete at best. I did have to try hard for my key accomplishments, but if you try hard too I am confident you will make it. I credit my physical therapy for my shocking accomplishments and would highly recommend all stroke survivors go to physical therapy for as long as possible (I will still go to physical therapy for at least two years and am in it now) and try their hardest (I often try so hard I break out in a sweat, but I do not sweat blood, like Jesus). Now, to those four accomplishments that fall just short of my list, but are worth mentioning, nonetheless.

On February 10, 2021, just five months after I suffered the strokes, I went in to work to get my first COVID shot. I would, subsequently, get a second shot and a booster at work too. Though this first shot was driven by real-world events (the global pandemic), I remember a shocking number of firsts about this event. I should start with my forty-mile commute to the office. That was, by far, the longest I rode in a car to that point. I remember parking in a handicap spot, but I still had to travel about one hundred feet to get into the building. I was using a walker at the time. It was also the first time I used my badge since the strokes. Every morning, I had to 'badge in' at turnstiles. The vaccinations were in the Auditorium, on the stage – usually a walk down about 20 steps without a railing to hold on to. I went the 'back way,' directly to the stage (though I did have to duck my head because of the low ceiling) – a handicap entrance.

The stage was a step up, and I could not do that at that time. I got some help up. The people giving the shots were very patient with me as I struggled to the raised stage. It turns out that actually getting the shot, probably a worry for almost everyone, was no big deal (by that point, I had gotten many shots, including in the stomach) – this one was in the arm. I have been in the Auditorium multiple times, and each time I challenge myself with some steps. I am happy to report at this time (the middle of March 2022); I can do about three steps and can get up and down the stage by myself. In fact, when I got my booster, I walked all the way up the stairs. But I digress.

Coming home that first time was a bit of a trip. First, I had to navigate my way off the stage. For some reason coming down is harder for me than going up. Always. But I managed to get down. I went through the hallway with the low ceiling again. Then, I had to walk through the turnstile. For some reason, with the walker, a voice always said I needed to go see security. This was the case when I went back to work too. Walking to the car was easy, and the long ride home was a piece of cake.

March 19, 2021, was my first day back at work. In those days, I was still using the walker (I would for a couple of months). It set off the turnstiles every time, and I thought I had done something wrong (so much was broken) until somebody told me they were on crutches and also set off the turnstiles. After that, I stopped worrying. Sure enough, they did not go off when I walked through the turnstiles without the walker.

In the beginning, I just worked five hours a day – just three days a week. The idea, which has been true to form as of this writing, was to build me up slowly. In those first few weeks back, I had a lot of expired training to do, and also had to get all of my Information Technology working, which proved to be a bit of a struggle. Predictably. There were also some new systems on which I needed to get certified. It was definitely, a busy period, with lots to do.

I also did physical therapy (PT), and occupational therapy (OT) exercises those first few weeks back at work. I guess the PT paid off, because I made the most progress there. So, I stopped doing the PT exercises at Christmas time (I would also do them at home). I had really surpassed them, but I still do the OT exercises to this day because they are designed to improve my reaction time, which will get me driving again.

On the physical side, I went on regular walks through the hallways and up and down the stairs of my building – without incident, and I got faster every time. I used to do the walks dating back to 2012 (when I was the captain of the team that won the ODNI pedometer challenge), and I still have the tee-shirt. I, basically, gamed the system and formed a team of people in training for marathons. I invented this walk then as a way to get the team more miles, and kept doing them after the pedometer challenge as a way to break up the monotony of the day. I tended to go with another person, though I sometimes went alone. It was a good break, and we have always talked about "work' on these walks. A lot of good ideas have come from them. So, we would go, together, on 'forced' marches. The walk is 0.8 miles. During the pedometer challenge, if I got all ten people on my team to go on the walk, well, that is eight miles.

On May 28, 2021, work threw a welcome back party for me. People, obviously, worked hard on it, as there was a lot of food, and a sign (which I am looking at now) welcoming me back signed by everyone with whom I worked. These events are a big deal in the Government, because they allow people to get away from their desks and blow off some steam. Some people get very involved and into it, and seem to enjoy cooking or decorating for everyone. My party was no different, and I greatly appreciated it. The best thing about my party was seeing old friends, several of whom came to the party. Kelly was supposed to come too, but, unfortunately, did not make it. The food-laden welcome back party is also useful to demonstrate my progress in 'carrying things.' I should also note that talking to your colleagues is a big part of these events.

As I said, these parties are fairly regular (~ every two months) occurrences for the government. The government celebrates most major holidays, and, I think some people enjoy cooking and decorating for their colleagues. Because these parties come along at regular intervals, like trolley cars, they were useful waypoints on my journey back. When I had the walker, my hands were full, but I could put 'dry goods' (like utensils) in a helpful basket Kelly got for me and attached to my walker. I was in a worse spot, despite having one free hand, with the waking stick because I had no basket and tended to hold the stick in my sound right hand. I was using the walking stick during my 'welcome back' party. When I started walking, I had two free hands and since the summer of 2021, see below, carrying food has been a significant story in my recovery.

When I started, with, probably, the 4th of July party, I was very tentative. We had practiced me carrying half-full cups of water in physical therapy, but I do not think those lessons were immediately transferred. When I started, I had trouble even carrying 'dry goods' in my right hand. Through time I got more confident and am now carrying full plates of food, or drinks, in my right hand and dry goods in my left hand simultaneously. Since this is a book about not being able to speak, it is important to note that at our Christmas Party, I 'sang' a verse of the twelve days of Christmas. The most recent get-together was to celebrate Mardi Gras, and I carried a full plate of food, with some gumbo, in my right hand, and in my left hand, I carried utensils and a roll. Most people do not think about what they carry at such get-togethers, but I do, and I am looking forward to carrying more at our St. Patrick's

Day Party – perhaps some corned beef and cabbage in my right hand and some soda bread in my left hand. I, like most people, will have to go back for the drink.

Finally, on July 4th, 2021, Independence Day, I gave up the walking stick and started walking. The timing was very contrived. I viewed, and view, walking as the sine qua non of Independence. Most people take walking around for granted. I know I did. DO NOT – it can be taken away from you in an instant by a freak accident, like with me. I know I will never take such things for granted again. My heightened appreciation for such things is a silver lining to this ordeal. Maybe I will celebrate Independence Day 2024 by driving (I will be almost 50), something else associated with Independence, which most people take for granted and I cannot do. I need ideas for 2022 and 2023.

My physical progress is truly remarkable as it is a yardstick of my overall progress. Moving from the walker to the walking stick and to walking without any support is very concrete. Nevertheless, physical progress hides my very real progress in other areas. I remain determined to progress in all things, tangible and intangible. I would highlight here two things; first, I would highlight 'words' generally, and second, I would also highlight my memory for song lyrics.

With words, I would point both to this book and a game I play on the phone. I feel like I have gotten stronger as I write this book, but you can judge for yourself (I, essentially, wrote Chapter 4 first, then the introduction, Chapter 3, Chapters 7, 6, 5 and 2, and then the conclusion. On my phone, I play Elevate (www.elevateapp.com) daily. Elevate is a competitor to Lumosity (lumosity.com), and I like it better, because Elevate works with my phone, whereas Lumosity does not. Margie, the speech therapist, turned me on to elevateapp.com, and I will almost certainly play it daily for the rest of my life. I play five games daily. Most of the games on elevateapp.com are synonym-based, and I set multiple high scores every day. So, it is the case that I am much better at math games than word games; I have always been this way. I tend to struggle, a bit, with new games I 'unlock' because it does take some time to get familiar with how a game works.

I always sang along to songs on the radio (or satellite, as it were) and knew the lyrics for thousands of Classic Rock and 'Contemporary' Songs. Well, I still sing along with songs in the car. Months ago, I found it quite difficult to sing along with songs on Sirus XM (we listen to channels 26, 25, 12, and the Beatles Channel). Margie said this would be the case, I think, because singers tend to go fast, but it is tough when you do not know what they are going to say. Although I will say, I have always found the slower songs easier. Over the past several months, more of the lyrics are coming back to me. I do not think this is due to hearing songs multiple times since my strokes, but, instead, I feel like this is coming from inside or 'upstairs.' I hope this trend continues because I enjoyed signing along greatly and would like to get back to it.

The Falling Trees

As I said, many of my biggest accomplishments occurred in late 2021 or early 2022. Figure 7 summarizes these events on a calendar, and it may be easier to visualize. While there is no word from my doctors, or therapists, on why 'firsts' should cluster a year or so from my strokes, it is certainly the case that the firsts are occurring faster and faster lately. Maybe there is some opportunity in the system, but I am a big believer that we create our own opportunities, and it is definitely the case that my hard work has created opportunities. One thing is for sure, if I can do these things, you can too; please use me as an inspiration. I will highlight thirteen events.

I am sure there are other firsts that I am not remembering, but these are big for me. I tried to produce as complete a list as possible. Some, no doubt, you will consider no big deal, like tying my shoes or shoveling snow, but to a stroke survivor using two hands (tying shoes) or strenuous physical activity with a real chance of slipping and falling (generally, shoveling snow) is a big deal. So, without further ado - to the list of achievements.

Sleeping Upstairs

The one event that fell outside the window was sleeping upstairs in my bed, which first occurred on November 15, 2020. It is not possible to overstate how huge this was, it made me feel normal. I remember when I first got home, and I was sleeping downstairs in the hospital bed, I could not roll over or do the stairs. It is a good indicator of the total destruction that I could not roll over at first. This was particularly frustrating because I am a stomach sleeper. In Encompass, generally, I was placed into a rolled-over position, and I really wanted to face away from the door because of the light in the hallway.

I worked hard in physical therapy (PT) to do the stairs. Practicing on the stairs was my favorite part of in-home PT. I remember first going up and down; I scared Kelly and my physical therapist (Megan) because I really wanted to go fast - I used to be an 'every other step' type of guy. This was the first time I had been on the stairs since August. It took me no time at all to master going up. Coming down, I was greatly aided by the banisters Ricky installed. It was not long, maybe the third time, before Megan wanted me to go "foot over foot," as she said. Basically, step on each stair with only one foot. Here, even going up, the banisters came in handy.

Now that I could do the stairs and roll over in bed, there was really no reason for me not to sleep upstairs. This was great both because it made me feel normal and because of the strange noises downstairs (what with the fish tank and refrigerator). Anyway, I slept much better upstairs and have been sleeping up there ever since. I think this event happened so early because both going up and down the stairs, and rolling over in bed are somewhat trivial, but I cannot overstate how huge this was for me.

I still, to this day, get 'caught' in sheets, and I disturb Kelly. The sheets tend to get caught under me, but I do not know why (I am asleep). I usually resolve the situation fairly quickly. The bigger disturbance is probably me using the bathroom, which I have to do at least once a night. Every time I get up, I also have to blow my nose (still like a trumpet). I feel like I wake almost everybody in the house up with that. I am also rumored to snore. I wear a breathe-right strip to bed to combat this, but usually take it off when I use the restroom. I have caught myself snoring a couple of times. It happens most frequently when I am on my back. Since I am a stomach sleeper, I am not on my back that much. I guess I snore loudly because the boys, clear across the house, can hear me. My Father used to vibrate the walls - I wonder if I do that? Anyway, it is how I express my love for my family, who must really be happy that I am sleeping upstairs.

Baltimore Aquarium

I remember when I went to the National Aquarium in Baltimore on March 29, 2021, I used the walker. Despite its help, we spent about two hours in the Aquarium and about thirty minutes walking around Baltimore's Inner Harbor, and it was a bit of a struggle. I got very hot, but I do not recall what I was wearing. Usually, if I expect to be warm, I wear something light. I really struggled on the long straightaways. There were some people in the Aquarium. The mass of people there did not bother me.

We went to the Aquarium as part of our Spring Break, where we stayed home. So, I went to the Aquarium, and Inner Harbor, and with my entire family. We ended the day by having dinner at the Hard Rock Cafe - where the boys devoured the food and did not notice the memorabilia on the walls. I noticed it, impressive. I used the restroom, at the Hard Rock Cafe, after dinner. I remember the restroom was down about 40 stairs. I discarded my walker and walked down and up those stairs with no problem.

I had been to the Baltimore Inner Harbor multiple times, so that familiarity helped. For example, the Fifth-Grade field trip every year was to Baltimore's Inner Harbor. I chaperoned every year. On that trip, we also went to Camden Yards (where the Orioles play if you live under a rock) to get a tour (that included going in the dugout and on the field) a big draw for me. I went on that trip each year the boys were in fifth grade. We also went to Baltimore's Inner Harbor as a family day trip about five times, and we visited Kelly's friend once and then walked around the Inner Harbor. We would also go to an Orioles game. I had also been to the Aquarium itself many times (at least five). It is famous and a great place for kids.

Nationals Game

We went to a Nationals baseball game on August 1, 2021. I went with my family, and this is the first of my cluster of events. I used to go to a lot of games, so this was a big deal. I went with the walker again, despite the fact I was walking, because of the long distances. The Nationals personnel and the other fans in attendance were very understanding. It was hot but tolerable as we were in the shade. We usually tried to get spots in the shade through the years, but that did not work every time. We got some expensive food and drinks. I continued my tradition of gathering large plastic cups. I went to the bathroom twice and tried to sing 'Take Me Out to the Ballgame' at the seventh-inning stretch. I prefer to sing America the Beautiful, but only the Yankees do this. They do so many things the right way. I used to make an annual pilgrimage to Yankees Stadium with the boys. I would like to get back.

I like to keep score at baseball games but did not keep score that day. I taught Timmy how; Ryan and Matty are not interested. I used to keep score while listening to games on the radio. I do not think there is a great deal of therapeutic value in keeping score at baseball games for me because this is something I did often. When I coached Travel, I would keep score in the dirt; in Little League, we had to have a dedicated scorekeeper. I think everybody should, at least, know the numbers of the positions. Ryan and Matty do, and I taught Matty's Little League teammates in the Fall. There is a lot of subtlety to keeping score a backwards K is a strikeout looking, and an IBB is an intentional walk, as opposed to a BB, which is a walk. I also liked to record where the pitches were by marking that in the scorebook. I used to keep score for Little League All Star games, when our Little League hosted the District Tournament. This is something I have done since my strokes and something I would like to do again. It is a great way to follow a game and a great way to recall what happened because you have a record. Keeping score also fights the tendency to not understand (see my favorite quote).

The Nationals games are great because kids can run the bases after games on Sundays. The line starts outside right field, and goes through the stands on the first base side. The kids start running at home plate, and run around all of the bases. Our boys have done this every season since they were three. A funny thing happened when the boys were seven, six, and three. Ryan, who was terrified by the Baltimore Oriole mascot when he was two, and held a grudge against large, inanimate creatures, punched Abraham Lincoln in the private parts as he rounded second. The Nationals mascots, the Presidents, occupied second and third base and home plate while the kids ran the bases. They gave the kids high fives. I have the image of Ryan rounding third, and Abraham Lincoln doubled over at second seared in my mind. By the time the boys were older, they had lapped many of the participants, who were little kids, not baseball players. I always wanted the boys to slide, at least into home, but we always went to summer Sunday games, and they were wearing shorts.

The Orioles are about as far from our house as the Nationals, and we would go to a bunch of games at Camden Yards. The Orioles have the benefit of playing the Yankees, and we would try to go to those games. Also, Camden Yards is a nicer ballpark than Nationals Stadium, so I prefer to go there. The food is, basically, the same, but the 'ambiance' is much better, plus I prefer the American League game to the National League. We have tickets, right now, to the Orioles and Yankees in April 2022, though the fate of this game is hanging in the lockout balance. I think they will play because the lockout is over. I did have to explain, to

Kelly and the boys, the differences between a lockout and a strike. This difference applies in all Labor Relations, and everyone should know this.

Plane Ride

On August 5, 2021, I went on a plane ride to Florida (about three hours). Traveling by plane was something I used to do often for work and with my family, and it was good to get back. We went to Disney. I used the wheelchair this time, mainly because of the distances at the park. I had not used the wheelchair in months, and the tires were flat on my ride. It was a struggle to pump the tires up, and Ryan pushed me. I also got stopped by the TSA for a 'pat-down,' which was odd because I was in a wheelchair and on the TSA exempt list (because of work). I guess I need to put my number on my forehead.

Parking at the airport was no big deal; I benefit these days from using the handicap parking spaces, we have a temporary pass. The bus ride at the airport was fine, and we definitely do not travel light. It was the same struggle as always getting on the bus, because of the bags. We have a bag per person. We have a lot of bags to check. I used to carry all the bags.

The plane ride went pretty well and was generally uneventful - like riding in the car. I brought plenty of stuff to read, like old times. I would read on the plane, and like old times, I also bought a College Football Preview Magazine at the airport. I got a window seat, like old times, and was comfortable on the plane. I also got some peanut M and Ms.

Traveling with my family is a production. We have to pack up the boys also and need to charge the screens to ensure they have something to watch on the plane. We download movies for the boys to watch on the plane, which is very important for Matty. I think we should go on more family vacations because these opportunities are diminishing. I mean, soon Ryan will be out of the house, to be quickly followed by Timmy. So, there are not many 'family' vacations left. Charged screens make plane rides and long car trips easy. We do not hear from the boys if they are watching screens - they generally keep their heads down.

The park was crowded, but okay. Kelly and the boys like visiting Disney. Kelly went as a girl; I think this is an important part of Americana for the boys. We got some recommendations on rides from my Bosses' Boss, who had recently gone with his family and is somewhat of a Disney aficionado. I tolerate theme parks, like Disney. They are hot and crowded, and I do not like the lines or rides. I have always been like this, even before the strokes.

Baseball Card Show

On November 27th, 2021, Thanksgiving weekend, I went to a baseball card show in Winchester, Virginia. I walked around for about an hour, and we spent cash on cards. Looking at all the cards on display was fun, but I feel sorry for the Dealers. Imagine (as I have often) if your profession was selling sports cards. When I was a kid, I would ride my bicycle to a store two miles away from my house. That guy who owned the store, nice enough, inherited the business from his mother. I spent hundreds of dollars there. From fifth grade on, I always had a job, and I spent all of my money until I met Kelly on sports, mostly baseball, cards.

I feel like most Dealers chose the profession of selling cards because they had to, and supplement their sports card sales by selling, also, fantasy cards (like Pokemon cards). I guess they need some annual income streams, like selling old baseball cards year around is not good enough. Dealers also need to keep abreast of all the latest varieties of cards, something regular guys like me can safely ignore. I have not gone for those new varieties of cards, dating all the way back to the late 1980s.

I enjoy bartering with the seller to 'talk down' the price listed on the card. We did a lot of this at the card show. The trick with baseball cards shows is that they have to be in your area, which for us, is about every six months. There is a big annual show in Baltimore, but we have never gone. We should - though I feel like Kelly has learned her lesson with me and baseball card shows. Expensive with me.

I dedicated a large portion of the second chapter to my vast sports card collection, but I am (and was at the time of my strokes) putting together the 1969 Topps baseball card set. I got about 40 cards for that set at the baseball card show. Not every dealer had those cards, so we had to look around. The cards I got can best be characterized as semi-stars (like Al Kaline and Carl Yastrzemski). The list price for the cards I got was about $475, so we 'talked down' more than $200. Kelly rejected my plan to get some more cards for Christmas.

Cutting Down A Christmas Tree

On November 29th, 2021, Thanksgiving weekend, we cut down a Christmas Tree. We go to a Tree Farm about fifteen miles from our house. We have always cut down a tree around then, at that Tree Farm. I always wonder, since a lot of people cut down trees at that Tree Farm and trees take a long time to grow, if the

Tree Farm ever runs out of serviceable trees. It was a bit muddy, but good to cut down a tree. I used to do the lion's share of the work, but did not last year. We got a local tree in 2020 (the Purcellville Volunteer Fire Department sells Christmas Trees as a fundraiser). I think the Fire Department must make a lot of money; they, generally, sell out in less than a week.

We also, generally, take a picture of the boys at the Tree Farm for our Christmas Cards. If not the Tree Farm, we take a picture of the boys around the house. This year we took a picture of them on the stairs. Kelly prints the envelopes for the Christmas Cards from a spreadsheet she keeps. We order the cards from Shutterfly. Judging from the Christmas Cards we get, many people do this. I stuffed the cards this year and was amazed at how many people on our list do not know about my struggles. I resolved to 'fix' this. I think I will contact the people on our Christmas Card list about this book. If the people on our Christmas Card list read this book, they will know (about my condition and a tremendous amount about me, maybe more than I would have liked before). Last year we did not send Christmas Cards; we had bigger fish to fry. I think, generally, if you do not get a Christmas Card from somebody you used to, something is up.

Going as a family and cutting down a Christmas tree is a nice tradition. I think the boys will carry this tradition on. Growing up, we had a fake tree. The stems and holes were color-coded to let you know where to put each branch, and there were about 30 semi-circle pieces for the trunk. Putting up the fake tree was as big a tradition as cutting down a real tree (and better for the environment). Either way, decorating the Christmas Tree is a nice family tradition. I have several decorations from when I was a kid, including some decorations my Mother made (she was very artistic). This year I helped decorate the tree and I helped take the decorations down. I did neither last year.

We also put out our Christmas Lights and put out Kelly's Christmas stuff. To say Kelly has a lot of Christmas stuff is an understatement (three huge bins full, other holidays have one, at times half full bins). Last year I could not help her. This year I helped with both. I need to help put up the lights because my height is an asset. Ryan is about as tall as me now, and can help, but he will only be around for Christmas 2022 and 2023. I really want to get a life-sized Nativity Set that lights up, but they are expensive, and I cannot find one I like. To say Christmas is a big deal in our house is an understatement.

Hotel Room

On December 1st and 2nd 2021, I stayed in a hotel room in Baltimore. I was there to see my neurologist at Johns Hopkins University, Dr. Rafael Llinas. This hotel stay was significant because the hotel room (shower) was a regular hotel room, not a handicap room. I can do a regular shower, thank God, it just takes all of my concentration. We used to stay in lots of hotel rooms, so staying in a regular hotel room this time was huge. It gives us a lot of flexibility. I should also point out that Llinas is the inspiration for this book. He suggested to me that I write it, and said that anything that made me think, at this point, is a good thing. Writing a book, certainly, makes me think.

Most hotels have breakfast in them, which is a big challenge, akin to carrying food at office parties. I can get my food (and make it; I always have a waffle). I am just really slow, and the other hotel patrons (who are getting breakfast too) are not witting to my condition. I usually get two plates of food and 2-3 cups of juice. I have to make three trips to the table to get it all. I fully take advantage of the free breakfast. Kelly also gets me tea.

Sleeping in hotels, regular rooms, or handicap rooms has historically been a challenge for me. I think, in the past, the weird noises bothered me. We tend to get our rooms from hotels.com and tend to be near the elevator. I also think that I did not like the strange bed. At any rate, I do not have any of those problems falling asleep (the strange noises and the new bed) in hotels now.

Wrapped Christmas Presents

On December 11th, 2021, I wrapped Christmas Presents. If you are a fan of specific, measurable progress, this one is for you because I could not wrap Christmas presents last year. I was never that good at wrapping Christmas presents, in fact, I pretty much sucked (I was very sloppy. I do not think I had the patience), but I would wrap for Kelly and add to the boys' Christmas lists and buy baseball stuff for the boys. I got back to these things this year and greatly appreciated them for what they are.

Last Christmas was very difficult for me because I could not do most things I wanted to do; it felt good to get back to some of those things this year. Wrapping Christmas presents for Kelly is a good example. Last year my left hand was simply not good enough to wrap. This year it was good enough for me to do a bad job. I also kept a detailed Christmas list for Kelly and contributed to the boys' Christmas lists... and bought one baseball thing, a new glove for Ryan.

I already have a Christmas list for Kelly for next year, so 2022, and have already gotten her three presents. I also have some good ideas for the boys. I am in the market for a Nativity Set. Typically, a trip would be among the boys' Christmas presents. I think we should go on another trip this year, we will see. Maybe not, because we already have one big trip planned. Timmy's birthday is right after Christmas, so we always try to get him a big present. In 2023 we are going to the Rose Bowl. Timmy should like that, and going to the Rose Bowl has long been on my bucket list.

Shoveling Snow

I shoveled snow, well-swept (global warming, you know) on January 7th, 2022. I used to shovel all the snow; Ryan and Timmy helped this time and all winter. I swept the path and steps to our house. Ryan and Timmy did the rest. To do our sidewalk, a neighbor used a snow blower (the equivalent of using a flamethrower to light birthday candles; nevertheless, I greatly appreciate it). This is very good because it is the law that you must clear your sidewalk within twenty-four hours of a snowfall ending. Kelly was very worried about me slipping, but I was not. I knew I would be careful, and I very much wanted to be out there. Also, Kelly is very cold and gets bundled up, whereas I am not that cold and do not need many clothes (I tend to sweat when I shovel or sweep the snow). Ryan is the same way and shovels in shorts.

I shoveled multiple times this winter and did more each time. I would get up to clean the cars and shovel the top part of the driveway. Next year I intend to shovel the entire driveway. I am getting ready for when Ryan goes to college, and that neighbor who used a snow blower on our sidewalk is moving. So, by winter 2024, I intend to shovel the sidewalk too. The sidewalk should be easier than the driveway (because it is flat). The real problem is the end of the driveway, which gets plowed in (if the plows come), and there is really no place to put the snow.

I always pay close attention to the weather forecast for snow. Actually, I am a bit of a weather buff. I guess it comes from coaching baseball and needing to know if it is going to rain, but I have always been interested in the weather. I am very interested in tropical weather too. I have never been able to understand people who were not interested in the weather, because it has such an outsized effect on people's lives.

I still read the National Weather Service's forecast discussion (they explain, well, what is going on). I also look at Jay's Wintery Mix on Facebook (Kelly likes him, as do all Northern Virginia Moms - he focuses on local weather and whether schools will close). I also look at tropicaltibits.com, which is great because you can play with all the models.

It is amazing how bad we are at forecasting what is going to happen with the weather. If you want to do a little experiment to drive this home, write down the forecast high temperatures for the next ten days and then record the actual high temperature. There will be a big difference. Weather systems are inherently chaotic, and this is particularly the case with snow (where we can only guess where the heaviest snow bands will set up frontogenesis, and can only guess if the two branches of the jet stream will phase, something that is important for our storms, and Nor Easters more generally). This has not been a waste of time for me. Weather models use Kalman Filters, a statistical model I have used in my work.

Tied My Shoes

I also tied my shoes, well boots, on January 7th, 2022. This may seem trivial, it is, after all, something we teach kids, but it requires two hands and is very difficult for me. I was actually afraid to try.

Necessity is not just the mother of invention; it is the mother of all things. I hate, have always hated, getting my feet wet when shoveling and wearing boots. Well, the last time, before January 7, 2022, I wore those boots was two years prior, and they needed to be tied.

My boots have two loops at the top of the foot that the laces need to go through before tying. The laces need to go through the loops in a criss-cross pattern. I did this, then I tied, double knotted, my boots. It took me a while (5 or 6 minutes) to do the first boot, but it took me about half that time to do the second boot.

My shoes and sneakers do not need to be tied, because the knots tend to stay (it is that way with double knots). I have, recently, undid the knots in my shoes and sneakers just to retry them, just for fun. I am warped.

Did 'the book' for Basketball

On January 15th, 2022, I did ' the book' for Matty's House basketball game. I did the book every other Saturday for the rest of the season. This is something I did hundreds of times before for the older boys - for both house and travel. For each game, two volunteers are needed, one to be the timekeeper (do the clock) and one to be the scorekeeper (do the book). If two do not show up at the table, the coaches go to the stands to get a volunteer per team. I always just showed up at the scorer's table.

Keeping score in a basketball game is complex work; you need to reconcile the score with the scoreboard at least every quarter. The hardest part of doing 'the book' is checking players in because you have to both look at the player to get their number and mark them in the book. It does not help that the players are anxious to get on the floor and tend to rush right by you. I can get some numbers while they are playing, though I have other things to do. There are minimum playing time rules in house, to which coaches must adhere, so keeping accurate track of who is playing is very important. The scorekeeper, 'doing the book,' must also record a coaches time outs (coaches get a maximum number of timeouts per half), and you also must count fouls per player (if they get five, they foul out) and the team. Per half (seven fouls total and your opponent is in a one and one and if you have ten fouls your opponent shoots two free throws). These last two team counts reset to zero in the new half.

It was good to be back, as I mentioned, this is something I did hundreds of times for the older boys. This year I did not do the clock, because you have to stop time immediately when the Referee blows the whistle and my reaction time is not great. That said, I practiced keeping time on my phone when I was not doing the book. One can anticipate some of the referee's whistles, but it is more difficult for whistles that occur during play, like fouls, tie-ups, and double dribbles.

African American History Museum

On February 17th, 2022, I toured the African American History Museum. I walked around for about three hours. There was a marked difference from the Baltimore Aquarium, more progress. In fact, I did not get tired or sweaty walking around - even on the long straightaways. I went to the Museum with work at that time and thank my Bosses' Boss (my former Reviewer), Damon, for walking around with me, and I should also thank Serena, who used to work for me, for walking me to the bus home. It is worth noting that I rode the bus there and back and read a book for work on the bus rides.

I would highly recommend the Museum, by the way, because it was well put together. They have both a lot of cool memorabilia, and the exhibits on the slaves are well done and moving. I kept a map of the Museum as both a memento and a reminder. It is amazing what they went through, and it explains a lot about the racial divide in this country. So, I plan to take the boys. It is vitally important they understand this history - it explains a lot.

It was great to be on the bus with people from work. The bus ride made me feel normal and demanded that I walk to our other office building, about half a mile from my former office. I had to walk back to my office after the bus ride. It was also great that people from work got to experience the Museum. We went as part of African-American history month. I hope my colleagues found the Museum as moving as I did.

Bowling

Lastly, on February 21st, Presidents Day, 2022, I went on a very special bowling trip. I organized a 'Trice Bowl' to mark the life and fondly remember my friend Andy Trice. He died from Pancreatic Cancer in 2017. I could say a great deal about Andy, he was a great guy, but I will only say three things about him here. First, he wrote a book about having cancer before he died and is somewhat of an inspiration to me. Second, he was big into the office esprit de corps. He organized many office get-togethers, like bowling outings. Third, one dimension of our friendship was daily trips to the gym. I think we both kept each other honest. A lot of good it did us.

We in the office did the Trice Bowl annually for about seven years and then fell away for three. I think both a reorganization and one of the prime movers behind the 'Trice Bowl' retiring caused us to lapse. The Government is forever reorganizing. The only constant is change. Gregg Burgess, who came up with many 'Trice Bowl' innovations, retired. Among Gregg's innovations included a handicap system that put everyone on equal footing and a 'Sandbagger' Award for the person who most outperformed their initial estimate. I have the winners' trophy from the last Trice Bowl. It was important to me that we restart, so, it was my idea to restart it.

I put together the invitation list, which was somewhat different than the historical list. Steve Heidorn took this list and transitioned it to an Evite. We included Andy's family this time and several Senior Executives from our old office. We also invited many of the participants from the olden days who showed up. This year's Trice Bowl was a big reunion. We did not invite one person who sued the Government in a case that went to the United States Supreme Court. Many of the other invitees had to testify for the government. It would have been too awkward.

Just conceptualizing the event, which we will now again do annually, was big for me. Putting together the invite list was even more important. It took a lot of brain power to figure out whom to invite, and whom to not. I used a ramp and kiddy bumpers. It was amazing to me how bad I got. I used to be good for about one-fifty. I was not a professional bowler by any stretch, but I was respectable. This time I rolled a seventy-five, a seventy-four, and a One-Fourteen. My ramp was definitely crooked, and I needed to adjust. I look forward to bowling like a normal human next year.

Conclusion

This chapter has been about some of my more stellar events since my strokes in August 2020. These events, certainly, had more to do with my physical progress than my inability to talk, yet I felt it was important to relay these events for two reasons. First, these events show people, or the loved ones of people, what can be expected about a year out. If I can do these things then anybody can. If I can be an inspiration to people, great. Second, these accomplishments demonstrate to my friends and family the value of my determination. It was through a sheer will that I accomplished these things. I was determined to do them, so they happened. It has been this way all my life. I will something to happen, then it happens. I am determined to drive and talk again so they will eventually happen.

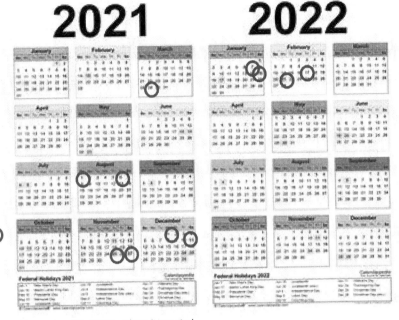

November 15, 2020 – Slept 'Upstairs'
March 29, 2021 – Baltimore Aquarium
August 1, 2021 – Went to a Nationals Game
August 5, 2021 – Plane Ride
November 27, 2021 – Went to a Baseball Card Show
November 29, 2021 – Cut Down a Christmas Tree
December 1-2, 2021 – Hotel Room
December 11, 2021 – Wrapped Christmas Presents
January 7, 2022 – Shoveled Snow
January 7, 2022 – Tied my Shoes
January 15, 2022 – 'Did the Book' for Matty's Basketball Game
February 17, 2022 – Toured the African History Museum
February 21, 2022 – Went Bowling

Figure 7: Accomplishments

CHAPTER 6
THE DAILY GRIND

What It Is Currently Like Being Me

This chapter will give you tremendous insight into what it is like being me, and my inability to talk is front and center (mostly). I start with a general overview, then go through my daily routine. There are some notable differences between weekdays and weekend days. So much so, in fact, I have a section for each, and because Saturday and Sunday are quite different, I have broken up those days.

So, you want to know what it is like living my life? The best I can describe it is that it is a little like being drunk all the time. I do not drink at all anymore; life is too short. I am what I was only more so, no fun too – with the twin frustrations of not being able to talk and doing everything slowly. The latter is a striking concern and, maybe, the topic for my next book, because I used to do everything fast (and still remember). It is very frustrating for me when I do a task and note how long it takes relative to how long it used to take. I deal with this now by keeping my frustrations internal and making mental notes of how to do things faster the next time. You should do this, or something better, too.

As far as being like I was, I was always a serial processor with unbelievable focus. Now, I can only do one thing at a time (kind of like forced serial processing), and I tend to hyper-focus on that one thing. I used to be very determined; now, I have a single focus. doctors and therapists agree that my determination will play to my advantage. Well, they have never seen anything like me. In fact, it is a goal of mine that the doctors will write books about the curious case of Kevin. I digress a bit. That is, after I am done shattering all the records. But, back to the chase. I used to get annoyed when the phone rang, because of the interruption; it was usually only spam anyway, but now I cannot talk on the phone. The 'do not call list' does not work. I was very in favor of plans – I used to say I would not go to the bathroom without a plan; now, I absolutely abhor spontaneity. I used to hate my commute and be constantly pressed for time.

In fact, I used to say I did not have time to wipe after I used the bathroom. This is life with young kids. I used to be highly competitive and have a difficult time trusting people. There is not much to be competitive about these days, but I really do not trust other people – who need to prove themselves to me constantly. It is a disease, I know, but it is one that not even two strokes could change. I think it comes from deep down and from being the first-born child of an alcoholic. I want to change but will probably go to my grave not trusting the undertaker. I used to take my faith seriously, but now, having almost died, I really take the afterlife seriously and believe wholeheartedly. Finally, I used to have a difficult time expressing my emotions. Nowadays, I cannot express my emotions verbally; they remain hidden. This is one way not being able to talk hurts most.

Being slow right now is like being stuck in a bad movie in slow motion. It is a movie because it seems like that through my eyes – like I am only, sort of, living it. Like a bad dream. The movie is bad because I have seen it before – it is my life, after all.

And I feel as if everything is in slow motion because it takes me roughly 200% longer than it used to, to complete the average task. But, again, it is very frustrating because I remember with total clarity what it used to be like. I wonder if there will come a time when I will not remember what it was like. Probably not, but maybe. The past will continue to haunt me.

On to my schedule, first, weekdays and then weekends. I present all in chronological order, with time stamps to help you.

Figure Eight gives you the layout of my bedroom. It will be helpful to review this figure before reading any further.

Weekdays

03:00 – I generally wake up at this time, or before, during the week and go over the plan for the day and the songs I will sing in the shower. I also need to use the bathroom; I have to 'go' much more urgently now. I think this is due to the strokes, not my age, because it happened suddenly and was correlated, in time, with my strokes. It is helpful to me to compartmentalize the plan for the day, and what I will say to Kelly when the alarm rings.

It is a little bit of a misnomer to say I cannot talk now; it just requires an unbelievable amount of preparation. I wonder if I will ever get to the point of being confident enough in my voice to go back to sleep when I wake up around 03:00 (which never fails, by the way).

The fact that I have to prepare so much really shows the effect of the non-fluent aphasia, from which I currently suffer. I have four groups now (my greeting for Kelly, the plan (which is everything) for the day, a random category, and a fourth category on the book. I have recently added the fourth category. I generally must write the plan for the day down to memorize it. We are like a 5-ring circus.

I wonder what I will talk about on weekdays when I am done with this book. Probably sports. It also takes me a few minutes to figure out what day it is, but it always comes. I am thinking about writing down my entire three, or four, category speech. I already write down the plan for the day.

I used to be very concerned with getting eight hours' sleep, but I do not care about that anymore. Whatever sleep I get, I get. I have noticed that if we have something the night before that taxes me or keeps me up, I tend to stay asleep longer before I am ready to go. This must be a common condition with strokes because my occupational therapist made mention of it. I recently read a book that opined stroke survivors need about 10 hours of sleep a day, so I take daily naps to make up the difference. I never used to take naps, saying they were for the weak. I guess I am kind of weak now.

05:00 – The alarm goes off. I try to turn it off quickly because I know Kelly does not like the sound (who does?). I have memorized how to turn the alarm off. Setting the alarm for the next day, especially if there is a different wake-up time, is a real challenge. I always set the alarm for the next day right then – something that was always the case. There is a different wake-up time on Fridays and weekends, and my alarm goes off in the morning, as the clock comes to the alarm time.

I do 7 stretches, which I recount here, because they may be useful to you. They are designed to stretch my tight hamstrings:

1. Laying on my back in bed, I pull my knees to my chest – 12 times each leg.

2. Laying on my back in bed, I raise a leg toward the ceiling; the stretch is greater if I point my toes to the wall – 12 times each leg. The 12 is significant for me. It is the number of repetitions the Loudoun Valley High School Baseball Team does in their workouts. I do this 'extra' too.

3. Laying on my back in bed, using the towel, I wrap the towel around my foot and raise my leg toward the ceiling, while holding the towel in my hands. I do this 3 times with each leg and say the "do-re-me" song twice and "take me out to the ballgame" once in my head.

4. Sitting on the edge of the bed now, I raise my knee toward the ceiling, in a marching-type motion. I say the "do-re-me" song in my head three times while I do this. There are 7 parts to the "do-re-me" song, so, I do this 21 times.

5. Also, sitting on the edge of the bed, I raise my leg (straight out towards the wall. This stretches my hamstring, more so if I point my toes straight up as I finish the stretch). I also do this 21 times because I say the "do-re-me" song in my head three times while I do this.

6. Also, sitting on the edge of the bed, I grab for the floor, while bending at my waist. I say the "take me out to the ball game" song in my head, so I do this 14 times.

7. Finally, again sitting, I rotate my torso with my arms extended. I also say the "do-re-me" song in my head while doing this. I go through the song 3 times, so, 21 rotations.

I do these stretches every morning – regardless of weekday or weekend, and will, almost certainly, do these stretches for the rest of my life.

05:30 – I shave. Kelly prefers me clean-shaven. She always has. Now, though habit, I guess, I really feel it if I do not shave, and so I try to do it every morning. I shave, even though this is very challenging for me, and I cut myself almost every day. It turns out my right hand is no bargain either in close quarters. I, generally, eschew the electric razor because it does not shave close enough. I leave a little bit of my face, and a little bit of the shaving. cream for my left hand. I feel, regardless of the cuts, I have made the most gains in shaving, and will continue to do so. I am very concerned, these days, with being clean-shaven. I wonder what I was like in the past – probably not as concerned. The hardest part for me is my chin, which never seems clean-shaven, no matter which way I go with the razor. I feel I will continue to get more efficient in this daily chore. The efficiency gains are likely to come both from shaving less (i.e., 'caring about being clean shaven' less) and from getting faster – nowadays, I tend to go over the same place multiple times. With shaving there is something to speed as you have to move the razor fast for it to shave.

06:00 – I shower. I shower left-handed (on the advice of Margie, she said it would help me) and sing in the shower. I am currently singing the "do-re-me" song (from The Sound of Music), "Take me out to the Ball Game", "Row, Row, Row your Boat", "Happy Birthday", and "Mary had a Little Lamb." I also say "buttercup" over and over (another trick from speech therapy, this one suggested by Elisabeth) and sing "The ABC Song" while walking down the stairs. I take requests. Buttercup was recommended by my speech therapist. You should try saying it over and over again; hard, is it not? I think she recommended it to me because it is a hard word with three syllables. Well, I say it four, then five, then six, up to twenty-five times in a row. When I think about how challenging showering with Nick was versus all the stuff I do now, it really underscores the progress I have made.

07:00 – My commute to work used to be about an hour. (Now on leave, I have replaced this time with doing a brian training game, and I have to email my former employer to "check-in" daily.) We used to listen to 'The Daily' podcast from the New York Times. I summarized each episode for Kelly, who drove me, from notes I keep. I have to keep, and read, the notes to make the words come out right. I tried doing it without notes, and doing so did not work out – another effect of non-fluent Aphasia, not being able to talk. The New York Times podcast is good because it keeps me up to date on current events, while the podcast is about one topic, each episode always ends with a rundown of the news headlines. I find its liberal bent somewhat annoying, but I do miss it. I also miss the sports podcasts I used to listen to when I drove. I had two good ones on the Yankees, and one on their AAA team (the Scranton Railriders), one on Ohio State sports (mainly football), two on the Islanders, and none on the (laughable) Jets. I also listened to the Bishop of Arlington, Hardcore History, Freakonomics, and a podcast on being happy (which was advertised on Freakonomics and was just starting out when I had my strokes). I have added a podcast on the weather.

08:00 – I arrived at work. I did the same three non-talking things every morning. First, I said good morning to about ten people on our instant messaging system. They did so much for me that it is the least I can do for them. Second, I used to clean my inboxes (I had three) of hundreds of emails. I got so many emails because I am on a lot of email distribution lists. One of my email systems was not working for a time – frequently was the case; we tend to have massive IT problems – government IT is the worst – probably because it is hard to get people to do IT and hard to get people to work for the government. Third, I forwarded a brief (for the Chairman of the Joint Chiefs of Staff and the Secretary of Defense) to some of my colleagues. I thought they would look for it anyway, but I hoped me sending it to them, and my commentary helped them. I also looked at the latest reporting and sent that out. I wonder if anybody does that now? I was on the distribution list for the Chairman's Brief brief for years. I used to rip the citations out of it. Distribution lists also tend to be sticky.

09:00 – I started my day at work. As I mentioned above, I believe I lost my job as a Group Chief because I cannot talk. A typical day was a blur of emails and meetings. I used to work four days a week but really wanted to go 'full time', that is, five days a week. Imagine that. My bosses were waiting for a report from some internal doctors who examined me, before giving me the green light to return to work full time. I worried about the validity of that report because I am constantly learning, growing, and changing, and the analysis was done in the early Winter of 2021… I wondered how/if that change would be reflected in that report. Going back to work 'full time' was one of the major issues in my life currently, and as I mentioned, I really wanted to do it (my doctors and therapists were all in favor, and so was Kelly). Working four days a week does offer me a degree of flexibility, which I liked. If I went five days a week, doubtless, I would give some hours back to the American Taxpayer, but this is what was happening before and is no big deal. We were only supposed to work 40 hours a week, 80 a pay period – which is two weeks. I used to work ninety or one hundred hours per pay period and was planning to return to that. I had more than enough work to support that, and the emails kept coming (like so many snowflakes).

Since going on leave, my days are filled with endless chores around the house, like doing laundry (we do about a load a day) and taking in the garbage cans. Doubtless, Kelly likes it, and it is good for my recovery. I also lift weights (we have free weights and a Universal Machine in the basement) and ride an exercise bike daily. These workouts are also good for recovery. Finally, I nap thirty minutes a day. I never used to nap, saying, "naps are for the weak," but sleep is proven to be important to stroke recovery (see Dr. Jill Bode Taylor, "My Stroke of Insight.") While I do all of this (even napping) I listen to some of those podcasts I missed.

16:00 – I typically ended my day around this point. I did the same thing every business day (I did this before, too) – I wrote down all my accomplishments for the day. It is a great practice, which I recommend that everyone does, and I really needed it now because I had trouble remembering, one day to the next, what I did. So, I mapped my accomplishments to the (ECQ)s – the Executive Core Qualifications put out for the United States Government by the Office of Personnel Management (OPM).

I still remember, when I was very junior, Sherry Barnes (my first supervisor), gave me a copy of the ECQs and told me I would be a Senior Executive someday. She was right, and I guess she saw something in me. I was driven to become a Senior Executive by the time I was 40; it shows you how competitive I was. Well, I made it at 43 and was close to my goal. The ECQs are publicly available and for SES (or SNIS) types. I was worried about the 'business acumen' ECQ because it is about managing people – something I no longer did. I wrote these accomplishments, and did the mapping, alone in my office, and doing so does not require me to talk. I cannot stress enough – everyone should do this, regardless of what they do for a living.

16:30 – I did my drive home. I started, in the same way, every business day. I walked out of my office, through the building, and down to the street. This was challenging because the area in front of the building is not level – I wonder if it is up to the Americans with Disabilities Act standards. The door to the building was automatic, a COVID thing, I think, and all you had to do to open the door was wave your hand. How I drove home differed somewhat. Kelly drove me home three days a week, and Kim Smith drove me home one day a week. Kelly picked me up right in front of the building. I had to walk to the top of the parking garage (which is fine) when Kim drove me. She parked on the top floor of the parking garage.

Regardless of who drove me home, I used to take advantage of the time - almost an hour, as I read and did brain training games (which I now do every morning). There was simply too much time not to take advantage of it. I have since replaced this time. Now I use it to work on this book and apply for new jobs. The job application process is both exciting and frustrating. It is exciting to apply for new jobs; one was to get paid to watch sports on television (well, you do have to write about the games). It is frustrating because you do not know if you are in contention for any particular job.

17:30 – I got home. It played the same way every weekday. I emptied my pockets and then went upstairs to take off my suit. All those things took much longer than they used to. I would highlight, as a particular challenge, taking off my suit. I could not wait until we went to business casual, as we were supposed to do. Taking off a suit was particularly challenging because of the many layers involved and the fact that some of what I am wearing (the socks, tee-shirt, and underwear) goes in the hamper in the bathroom, and some of what I am wearing (the suit, shoes, tie, and belt) goes in the closet. So, unless the suit needed to go to the cleaners, about every three 'wearings,' and I have seven suits, so, it works out suits go to the cleaners about once a month. I have never sent my ties (I have about fifty) or my shirts (I have about a dozen) to the cleaners.

There is a separate spot in the bathroom for my shirts, which we launder. I tend to put on sweatpants and a sweatshirt – a marked difference from the suit and probably a relic from my coaching days. These days not having to take off a suit is a relief and a big time saver.

18:00 – We eat dinner at this point. We try to eat dinner together, as a family every night, but extracurriculars interrupt. We start with grace. We try to eat good food, but Matty is very picky and will only eat certain foods – mostly junky-type foods. He reminds me of me, very particular in what he eats. Kelly always cooks dinner with the food we buy on Sunday. Eating, for us, takes a lot of planning. Dinner is uneventful for me; I can get all the food in my mouth. I am frequently reminded of the cafeteria at Encompass. When I eat, I mostly use my right hand. I usually have water with dinner, and I do not drink that much of it for fear of going to the bathroom at night. This is very different from what it was before the strokes when I tended to have a large cup of water. I have a collection of cups, the 32-once variety, from sports stadiums and various games I have been to. I would hang out a bit after the game and pick up cups left by others. Prized are the cups from far away, exotic stadiums. We have cups from the San Francisco Giants and Pittsburgh Pirates. We have a lot of cups from Ohio State and the New York Yankees. I cannot wait to go to Ohio State, Yankees, and far-flung games again. I have been to most major league cities to see games at this point, I have also been to a World Series game at Yankee Stadium (a bucket list thing) I have the ticket stubs (when we used to get tickets) and cups – to prove it! I wonder what Rose Bowl cups are like?

Before, I was not too concerned with going to the bathroom because I sweat a lot in the evening as I was usually outside, coaching baseball, and throwing batting practice. I have holes in my socks, "Holy Socks," to prove it.

I also used to talk a lot during dinner, and try to get the boys to talk, but I do not (cannot) do that now. This stinks and is the worst effect of non-fluent Aphasia.

19:00 – My post-dinner routine currently involves watching the NBC Nightly News, which we tape on DVR so we can fast forward the commercials. I feel like everyone does this, and they should not make commercials anymore. I can tolerate NBC News because it is, mostly, straight and does not have any opinion in it. I want somebody to tell me the sky is blue, not why blue is their favorite color. I prefer to make up my own mind about world events. The big story now, to date this Chapter, is Russia invading Ukraine. I think Putin did it because he knows NATO, and the United States, will not do anything militarily. Just economic sanctions, which may or may not work. This was a big debate on sanctions effectiveness when I left Academia. I really do not want Lester Holt's opinion about the matter.

20:00 – At 8:00 pm, I have my medication. At night I take Melatonin. Melatonin is in chewable, tasty form. I have two chewable doses, 10 milligrams (a double dose), because it tastes so good and will not hurt me. I wonder why the Melatonin does not help me stay asleep? I have a powerful incentive to wake and stay awake.

20:30 – I typically go to bed around this time. I think if I stayed up later, I would sleep later. I say my prayers and have no trouble falling asleep. As I said above, I am a stomach sleeper, and

I usually fall asleep when I get into this position. It is like clockwork.

Saturdays

The weekend is different in four notable ways: First, we sleep later. Second, I cut the hair in my ears and nose (I have to do this daily now). Third, I have been recently getting my own breakfast and lunch. Fourth, we change our sheets and towels, a valuable habit. Getting my own breakfast and lunch on Saturdays is a major step forward because I did this before my strokes. I also have a can of Diet Coke on the weekend. I used to drink three cans a day, and it is great that I am drinking some of it on the weekend, because it gives me something to give up for Lent. We also all tend to give up desserts. Easter Sunday, with all its candy and deserts, is much more special.

03:00 – I tend to wake up around the same time and do the same things as during the week. One notable difference is that I usually must go to the bathroom twice because of the later wake-up time. This is a shame, I wish I could take advantage of the later wake-up time, but I cannot. The forces are just too powerful.

06:30 – The alarm goes off; the same things tend to apply as during the week.

06:30 – I shave. It is like during the week with one notable difference. I have always (well, as long as I can remember) cut the hair in my ears and nose. I think of this as, kind of, a tax. I expect these hairs will grow faster as I age and I will have to trim this hair more often. Notably, I resisted the people who cut my hair cutting my eyebrows because I am a firm believer in, 'if you cut it, it grows.' Recently, I have let them cut my eyebrows, and I have added this to the Saturday morning routine.

07:00 – I shower, and on Saturdays, I change our towels. Kelly usually changes the bedsheets and blanket. The new towels/bedding is located in the upstairs hallway, so not too far. I would recommend you get into a regular pattern like this – it will ensure you always have a clean towel and sheets.

08:00 – We eat breakfast. Saturday breakfast in our house is a big deal, and we eat as a family and have panckes and meat. We also have hamburgers and hot dogs for dinner every Sunday night. Since Ryan was born in 2005, we have had an unbroken streak of having pancakes (or waffles) and bacon (or sausage) for breakfast on Saturdays. Kelly always cooks and makes pancakes (or waffles) from scratch with a recipe and raw ingredients. This has been regardless of what else has been going on – and there have been times when we had a lot going on. Kelly and I are big believers in kids thriving with consistency, which is one bit of consistency we have brought to Ryan, Timmy, and Matty. So, it will be interesting to see if we continue the streak when our nest is empty; I like having a 'special' breakfast on Saturdays too.

I also eat an apple every day. Doing so is supposed to keep the doctor away. Unfortunately, that did not work out for me, but I like apples (Gala), which has become part of my daily routine. We also try to make the boys eat fruit. Timmy will eat some, but Ryan and Matty will not. All three boys have yogurt and apple juice every morning (along with two gummy vitamins). More consistency.

10:30 – The boys have some sort of sports practice on Saturdays – we are not off on the weekends. There is always a lot going on. It is important to note here two things. First, I was often the coach for the boys, so, not off. Second, this is how kids play now. Gone are the days of playing with the kids 'on the street.' All playing time is now scheduled. I have never been able to decide if this is a good thing. On the one hand, as the coach, I was really in my kids' lives. On the other hand, there is a value to free play.

12:00 – We eat lunch. We tend to eat as a family on both days. We usually have sandwiches (we go through a lot of cold cuts) and potato chips (or pretzels), and, as I mentioned, Kelly is now making me get my own, which is fine – lunch is typically uneventful. Here I will mention what I cannot do (and what Kelly still does for me):

1. I really struggle to carry full glasses (usually of water, though Cranberry Juice with Breakfast). We worked on this in PT, but, I guess, not enough. It is important to note I have a lot of juice in the morning, typically a full 32 once cup. This is as it was before, I am thirsty in the morning.

2. Kelly gets me fruit in the morning. It comes from a plastic jar and goes in a bowl. I think I can do this; it is probably just a habit for her.

3. Kelly makes me eggs some mornings. I would struggle to break eggs. I used to not like eggs, but they are easy to eat (and we had them often at Encompass), nutritious, and tasty. The juice, water, and eggs are just waiting for me.

4. Kelly also makes me tea in the mornings. We are tea drinkers, always have been. She drinks her tea hot. I like (and liked) to wait for it to cool down, and then chug it. I have always disliked hot beverages.

Come to think of it, this is all breakfast stuff, and I am good to go for lunches.

13:00 – Lately, I have been working on the book, but this is primetime for college sports on Television. I really watch Ohio State but will watch anybody (and root for a close game) and any sport. In this way, Timmy is like me; he will watch anything. My favorites are football and 'Winter' sports. I like watching the Olympics. For those competing in those sports, the Olympics is the culmination of a lifetime of hard work. I appreciate that and like the 'exotic' nature of winter sports. I wish the United States was better at them. I tend to DVR most games, so I can fast-forward the commercials and watch them on the weekends. I have discovered that you can watch baseball and football games on fast forward. This has the benefit of muting the play-by-play, which I find annoying. I know what is happening. Sometimes the color commentary is okay, but more often, it, too, stinks.

18:00 – We eat dinner; this is like during the week except that we usually get take out on Saturdays. There are entire restaurants that Matty does not like, and he tends to get pizza (the kid is made out of pizza) or grilled cheese sandwiches. Same as during the week, I tend not to drink that much with dinner on Saturday. We never get drinks with take-out. It is a waste of money, and we have drinks at our house.

19:00 - My post-dinner routine is just like the week. I watch the DVR of NBC Nightly News – if it is on (sometimes it is not because sports ran late). The DVR does not know, and we usually get a tape of the end of whatever games were on.

20:00 – I have the same pills as during the week; medication is a constant.

20:30 – Just like the week, I go to sleep. Though, sometimes, I stay up a little later. We tend to have 'family movie/TV nights' on Saturdays and used to watch 'Batman.' That show is ridiculous, but it is an important part of Americana that the boys must know. I also subjected the family to watch 'Gilligan's Island' - for the same Americana reason. I have a DVD of all 'Gilligan's Island' episodes and find it very relaxing to watch, even though I know what is (not) going to happen.

Sundays

03:00 – I tend to wake up around the same time and do the same things as during the week and go to the bathroom twice. I also go over the same sorts of things in my head.

06:30 – The alarm goes off, and I do my stretches – like during the week. I tend to hurry, because we have a lot to do on Sunday.

06:30 – I shave. It is like during the week.

07:00 – I shower, same as during the week. There is nothing special about Sunday, though I do try to hurry. Sunday gets really nuts when there is a travel baseball doubleheader or an out-of-town tournament. We tend to re-arrange our schedule for those. I used to coach those. I have no idea how we fit it all in.

07:30 – Kelly, usually, eats and puts together the shopping list while doing so. We consume a tremendous amount of food, and Sunday is usually our last chance to go to the grocery store for the week, so this is huge.

07:45 – I write out the checks for church. Though we could give electronically, Kelly and I feel there is a valuable demonstration effect for the boys of us putting envelopes in the collection basket. So much so, that I used to make the boys put the envelopes in the baskets themselves. I have been doing the checks for months, I used to do the checks, and little did we know it, but writing checks was on a test the doctors at work gave me. So, the practice helped.

08:00 – On Sundays, I tend to scarf down what is around for breakfast, though I usually add cereal and toast (buttering the toast is a challenge for me). To my juice (which Kelly leaves for me at my spot at the table) and an apple. I look over the readings for church while I eat. I now have a Lector Workbook, and I tend to look there.

As an aside, I am planning for the day when I will be Lector again. I am shooting for Ryan's last Mass as an Altar Server (which will happen sometime in the summer of 2023). Lector will require me to get my voice back, which I am working on (see below), and will also require me to walk up and down, three steps without a railing. On the latter, I practice at home (though we have railings, I do not use them on the three steps that lead to our house), and I have been, recently, practicing on the Altar itself at Church. I do this after Mass, like a ghost, and I also pay close attention to what the Lector has to do – there is much more to know than just the readings.

A tip from Margie (my former speech therapist) for public speaking is to put little lines in the text where you will take breaths. I do this with a pencil, just like I am going to Lector. This is important, as we shall see.

It is currently the case that Kelly also gets the boys up around this time. They all have some form of CCD (Confraternity of Christian Doctrine), on Sundays at 09:00 and need to eat. They typically wander into the kitchen, none too happy to be up. I make them wear black shoes and pants, in case they have to serve. When the boys are scheduled to serve, they must wear black pants and shoes. It is frequently the case, like once a month, that the other Altar Servers do not show, and our boys are pressed into service. There are four roles for Altar Servers currently, but both of our Priests have said they do not care how many Altar Servers there are. So, theoretically, Ryan, Timmy, and Matty can serve every week. Studies have found that more than eighty percent of Priests were Altar Servers, and I would be okay with one of our boys 'taking one for the team.' Ryan has always been my candidate; he has the demeanor of a Priest and is very altruistic – a key personality trait for Priests. That said, I have difficulty envisioning Father Ryan.

09:00 – The frantic time. The boys go to CCD and Kelly and I go food shopping, usually in a rush. Ryan and Timmy have been Confirmed (Eighth Grade) and help out with teaching; Matty is currently in sixth grade. I used to do the grocery shopping by myself but cannot anymore since I do not drive. Kelly has always done the shopping list. We use two huge bags to carry the groceries (it is just more efficient), and I (for months) push the cart around the grocery store. I find, and have found, it remarkably easy to push the cart around. It gives me something to hold onto. We bring those bags and the list with us to the grocery store, and Kelly and I rush around the store (the boys are done at 1015), grabbing the mounds of stuff on our list. Of note, the boys consume gallons of apple juice and milk per week, and we stock up on Sunday.

We fill both those huge bags and then some (usually) and head home to unpack. Despite the two huge bags, carrying the groceries into the house is hard. I cannot take the large bags, and Kelly struggles to lift them (they weigh about 50 pounds). I have been practicing taking the large bags in recently. I desperately want to help Kelly. I will probably be able to carry both big bags after the boys leave the house - there will be no more need for big bags; I cannot eat that much. Once we lug the groceries in, we have to put them away. My slowness really hurts us. Sometimes we cannot even put the groceries away before we have to get the boys, but we usually do, so, I will write about that case.

Kelly puts most of the stuff away, and I try to help. Usually, I end up just breaking boxes. I also replace the pretzels (we go through a bag a week) and my apples. Both involve plastic bags – which we recycle. We also use the restroom.

We have to supplement this haul with a monthly trip to COSTCO, where we fill a cart, always. The trip to COSTCO follows the same script – Kelly list, Kevin cart. I never used to go to COSTCO, but I enjoy it now (well, as much as one can enjoy such things).

10:15 – We must be at the Church to get the boys. I read aloud the readings for the day in the car on the way to Church. Sometimes I wait until the boys are in the car. I think it is important that the boys hear the readings and think about them before Mass, which is really good practice for me. The lines I put in the text are helpful, though I always want to get more words in before I take a breath – a bit of a hangover from when I was a Lector, I think.

10:30 – We go to Mass as a family. Always. I believe you have to be dead to miss Mass (and, even then, you get one). For the longest time, we were sitting in an easy spot for me, but we have returned to our customary pre-stroke position in the pews. Kelly got me a Daily Missal, which I use to follow along, but I find it challenging to keep up with the prayers in the Mass. I also try to sing and am thinking about joining the choir. I think this would be great for me. I was signing in Mass before my strokes. St. Augustine said singing was like praying twice. I keep waiting for the day when I can keep up; I try really hard and believe that day is coming and I will be ready.

12:00 – We eat lunch. We also tend to eat lunch as a family on Sunday, though the boys are in a strange mood after CCD and Mass. Like Saturday, we usually have sandwiches (we go through a lot of cold cuts) and potato chips or leftovers. I, generally, try to eat the leftovers if we have them. I pride myself on 'thinning the herd' in the refrigerator. Kelly is now making me get my own, which is great progress.

13:00 – On Sundays, by 1 pm, we tend to revert to what to other 99% of the population is at this time – relaxed. At this time, I should make special reference to NFL Red Zone – the greatest thing since sliced bread, seven hours of commercial-free football. If you do not have it, you should get it. It is constantly on in our house during football season – a host flips between games and tells you what is going on. They are really on top of things and show every scoring play. Timmy likes it too. It is a must for Fantasy Football players.

13:00 – We mow and weed whack the lawn during the spring and summer. I do one side, and the boys handle the other side, front, back, and weed whacking. I can do it all, but it takes me four to five hours.

15:00 – I usually practice driving on Sundays at this time, in a parking lot by some baseball fields I used to frequent. I drive fine in straight lines, and there is a curve and a stop sign on which I practice, but keeping my hands at '10' and '2' (well, 8 and 4) and doing 'mirror, mirror, blind spot' all the time is a bit difficult for me. I used to drive, often, with one hand, so '10' and '2' is particularly challenging. I also practice parking, and there are a bunch of parking spots there. I can pull into a spot on the driver's side, no problem. I have a little trouble pulling into a spot on the passenger's side. We have not practiced parallel parking, and I never once used that skill in all my years of driving. I also practice going in reverse. I still remember all the traffic rules and have a habit of texting them to Ryan (who is driving now). I find this helpful, and it is great to practice, but I really want to get driving on the road again. The big hang-up for Kelly is my reaction time, which, unfortunately, is impossible to simulate in the parking lot, but I do (daily) some games for reaction time that Laura turned me on to. We return to find Timmy where we left him, and he updates me on the games. I, generally, return to watching Red Zone, with a brief interlude to get my clothes out for Monday.

16:00 – Kelly usually talks to her parents. These chats are important to her sanity and her parents, John and Sue, typically have some good ideas for me.

18:00 – We eat dinner, this is like during the week except that we always have hamburgers and hot dogs for dinner on Sunday. More consistency. I tend to help nowadays by setting the table and getting out the buns. I used to be coaching at this time of day and could not help. Kelly cooks the dinner with corn, and fries (or onion rings, my favorite, Ryan eats them too, but Timmy and Matty do not). We are forever planning meals around the various peccadillos of our kids.

18:30 – Ryan and Timmy have Youth Group, and Matty (sometimes) has MAC-PAC (Middle Schoolers Acting for Christ: Prayer Action Charity). I think they have an on again, off again, meeting schedule because they are so young.

19:00 – Red Zone ends by showing every touchdown from every game… I look for Buckeyes (it is usually Ezekiel Elliot or Terry McLaren who score these days). I used to ice my knee at this time but do not have to anymore because I am not throwing batting practice.

20:00 – Like during the week, I have my medicine.

20:30 – Like every other night, I go to bed. Sunday night was important because Monday brought work. If I did not do so already, I put out my clothes, shoes, and socks for the next day. I have always done this anal behavior.

Conclusion

I would conclude by saying that my condition preventing me from talking does not affect most chores in my day, but when it rears its ugly head, it has a significant effect. This rearing happens most often formulating the plan for the day; it affects my sleep, for crying out loud, summarizing the podcast, and at the dinner table – where it hurts a lot. I can communicate now, in real-time, with facial expressions, but this method is not optimal because it is easily misinterpreted.

But like above, its effect is only moderate – on some things. I have a lot of daily solitary tasks that do not require talking. So, I guess this is good. I am learning writing this book that my not being able to talk does not have as big of an effect as I thought, and I plan to talk again.

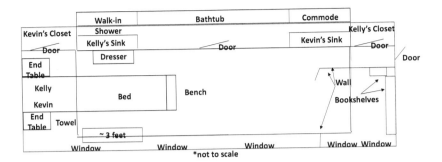

Figure 8: My Bedroom

CHAPTER 7
THE 4 LESSONS

This period has sucked, but there have been silver linings - my sons have definitely learned at least four big lessons during this ordeal: First, from me, they learned that human life is fragile. Second, also from me, they learned the value of determination. Third, from Kelly, they learned what one spouse should do for another. The vows do say, "in sickness and in health." Fourth, from Kelly again, they learned what a 'Super Mommy' can do when she puts her mind to it. No doubt, the most powerful force in the Universe. I love my sons more than words can say, and would lay down my life for them; what father would not? It is beyond great that we have been able to teach them some valuable lessons, so at least something good will come out of this situation. In this chapter, I will detail each of the lessons and conclude with the value of struggle. Along the way, I will count my blessings (something we should all do), then briefly talk about Church.

It is the case that none of these lessons have to do with my inability to talk; in fact, my various maladies (inability to talk included) have really helped drive these lessons home. There is really a lot for which to be grateful. I am reminded of Pope, Saint John Paul the Second, who said his suffering later in life was a blessing. Mine too. A little bit about a great man... When he became Pope in 1978, he was an avid sportsman, but during his 26 years as Pope, he declined, and near the end of his life, he developed Parkinson's Disease. He developed many maladies too, and even had difficulty speaking more than a few sentences at a time. He also had trouble hearing and severe osteoarthrosis. Despite all of this, he continued his practice of touring the world (he visited 129 countries).

The first lesson my sons learned is on the fragility of human life. They learned this lesson from me. When I was their age and into my 30s (despite Matt), I thought I was indestructible. Well, I (we) was (are) not. I was Super Daddy, King Supreme, and doer of all things. To see me fighting for my life with all sorts of tubes coming out of me and in an intensive care unit (ICU) must have been quite a shock, but it underscores that all human life is fragile – if this previously indestructible force of nature could be reduced to almost nothing, well, that is a powerful lesson. To learn it at such a young age: 17, 15, and 12 is a real gift (ages now, ages at the time: 15, 13, 10). It also underscores for me, by the way, that I should be thankful for every single day – something, objective-oriented me, has historically struggled to realize.

For example, I now value every day (I did not before). I also do not get angry with my kids as frequently. Finally, I now see beauty in all things.

The second lesson my sons have learned is also from me – the value of determination. Determination is the most important key to success as we often fail. Interestingly baseball, which they all play, or played, is also about failure (see the Ted Williams quote in Chapter 4, this applies to all endeavors). I have already demonstrated that one can overcome obstacles through determination and when I lick this thing, I will really demonstrate the value of determination. Usually, even now, I fail on my first try, produce a mediocre effort on my second try, and tend to get things right on my third try.

For example, I mastered the stairs and went from a wheelchair to walking on my own. Both took real determination. In fact, I usually try things repeatedly until I get them right. This stick-to-it-iveness was a hallmark of my previous life and is true today. With each task I complete, I demonstrate the value of the most important human quality, effort, to my sons. I have a saying that bears repeating here; success = skill*effort. You cannot control skill; that is God-Given, but if you always try your hardest, no one can fault you for lack of effort, and you will, probably, succeed.

The nuclear family (Father, Mother, Kids, under one roof) is the most powerful institution in the world and the third lesson my sons have learned from my wife Kelly, is what one spouse should do for another. Kelly has done everything for me and, in so doing, has demonstrated this lesson to our sons. The Wedding Vows do say, 'in sickness and in health,' and I have been very sick. Kelly has taken care of me because it is the right thing to do, and I would do the same for her. Actions are more important than words, and Kelly has really shown this virtue to our sons. One cannot overstate how important this is for me. I loved her before and will love her forever now. We will probably, haunt our sons when we are gone – if we can.

Fourth, the boys have learned what a 'Super Mommy' can do. Kelly has done everything, including taking care of me and shuttling the boys around for their busy extracurricular schedule, and in so doing, has demonstrated the most powerful force in the universe – that of Super Mommy. Mothers are said to lift cars off their trapped children, and I really believe it from what I have witnessed. I hope the boys always fondly remember their mother. What Kelly has done, in this trying time, ought to guarantee that.

1. Fragility of Human Life
2. The Value of Determination
3. What one Spouse Should do for Another
4. Super Mommy, The Most Powerful Force in the Universe

Kevin   Kelly

Figure 9: The 4 Lessons

From our boys, we have definitely learned resilience. Despite my situation, they have continued to excel in all aspects. They could have totally fallen apart, but they have not. They continue to do well in school (almost all As), succeed in sports, volunteer at church, and get up every morning ready to face the day. They are great and very resilient, some would say determined.

For example, Ryan did great when he took over the Fall Little League team from me and really helped me coach this past Fall. Plus, he has done well in school. Matty and Timmy have also helped me around the house and have continued to rock school. No Cs are allowed for the Sweeney boys (see my bit about effort above), and it really does not matter – they get all As, and I am very proud of them.

The Value of Being Properly Thankful

I think everyone should know the value of being thankful and keeping a gratuity journal; the effect on you is real, so I quote one study at length here:

"About three months after the psychotherapy sessions began, we took some of the people who wrote gratitude letters and compared them with those who didn't do any writing. We wanted to know if their brains were processing information differently.

We used an fMRI scanner to measure brain activity while people from each group did a "pay it forward" task. In that task, the individuals were regularly given a small amount of money by a nice person, called the "benefactor." This benefactor only asked that they pass the money on to someone if they felt grateful. Our participants then decided how much of the money, if any, to pass on to a worthy cause (and we did in fact donate that money to a local charity).

We wanted to distinguish donations motivated by gratitude from donations driven by other motivations, like feelings of guilt or obligation. So, we asked the participants to rate how grateful they felt toward the benefactor, and how much they wanted to help each charitable cause, as well as how guilty they would feel if they didn't help. We also gave them questionnaires to measure how grateful they are in their lives in general.

We found that across the participants, when people felt more grateful, their brain activity was distinct from brain activity related to guilt and the desire to help a cause. More specifically, we found that when people who are generally more grateful gave more money to a cause, they showed greater neural sensitivity in the medial prefrontal cortex, a brain area associated with learning and decision making. This suggests that people who are more grateful are also more attentive to how they express gratitude.

Most interestingly, when we compared those who wrote the gratitude letters with those who didn't, the gratitude letter writers showed greater activation in the medial prefrontal cortex when they experienced gratitude in the fMRI scanner. This is striking as this effect was found three months after the letter writing began. This indicates that simply expressing gratitude may have lasting effects on the brain. While not conclusive, this finding suggests that practicing gratitude may help train the brain to be more sensitive to the experience of gratitude down the line, and this could contribute to improved mental health over time.

The GGSC's coverage of gratitude is sponsored by the John Templeton Foundation as part of our Expanding Gratitude project.

Though these are just the first steps in what should be a longer research journey, our research so far not only suggests that writing gratitude letters may be helpful for people seeking counseling services but also explains what's behind gratitude's psychological benefits. At a time when many mental health professionals are feeling crunched, we hope that this research can point them—and their clients—toward an effective and beneficial tool.

Regardless of whether you're facing serious psychological challenges or if you have never written a gratitude letter before, we encourage you to try it. Much of our time and energy is spent pursuing things we currently don't have. Gratitude reverses our priorities to help us appreciate the people and things we do." (Brown and Wong, 2017)[16]

I keep a gratuitry journal and write a lot of thank you notes (about one every other day). I think it would also be appropriate to count my blessings here. People, generally, do not do that, and being grateful has been scientifically shown to have a positive effect on your well-being. In fact, I was encouraged in a course on Leadership at (Gulp!) the University of Michigan to keep a gratuity journal. You should do the same. You write down, each day, what you are grateful for, and there are no wrong answers. I started doing this, then stopped. This is a practice I should start again.

I am grateful for the following:

1. The Boys and Kelly are healthy, as are our extended family and friends.

2. Kelly and I have enough money and a comfortable house in which to live.

3. Kelly has a great job with a great boss.

4. I have great medical insurance.

5. I have plenty of leave, which I am now using.

6. We have two cars that work.

7. We, mostly, eat healthy, and we have enough to eat.

---

[16] Brown, Joshua and Kolton Wong. 2017, "How Gratitude Changes You and Your Brain," accessed online (January 23, 2023): https://greatergood.berkeley.edu/article/item/how_gratitude_changes_you_and_your_brain

8. I am grateful for my determination, focus, and drive – elements of my success.

9. I am grateful that I have strong faith and rest assured in the Resurrection.

10. I am grateful that I am a Yankees fan, and they usually win.

11. I am grateful that I am a Buckeyes fan, and they usually win.

12. Being a Jets, and recently, an Islanders fan has been great for my sense of humor and humility.

13. I am grateful I am a Catholic, see a miracle every Sunday, and am assured of resurrection. St. Thomas Aquinas said, at the resurrection we would all be about 33 years of age. That would be fine with me, though Matty did not exist yet when I was 33, because I was healthy.

14. Specific to my situation, Ryan has decided to pursue physical therapy as his life's work. I view this as a great compliment, as my physical therapists have really helped me. I am further grateful that both Ryan Cusack and Helen said yes when I asked them to mentor him. I always thought Ryan would be a Priest, he certainly has the temperament for it, but this is better.

15. Specific to my situation, I am grateful for all the doctors, therapists, family members, and friends who have taken care of me. I deeply respect friends - I have lots. There are some advantages to being oversubscribed.

16. Specific to my situation, I am grateful I lost 15 pounds. It is one of the great ironies of my life that I slaved away, very early, in the gym at work and did not lose any weight. I guess I had to have strokes to lose the weight.

17. Specific to my situation, my teeth are much better. It is impossible to overstate what a mess my mouth was/is. I have more crowns than the Hapsburgs. This is one way Encompass really helped me. I now floss twice daily and use mouthwash in the morning. I picked up both habits at Encompass. I also stopped chewing gum, which was a near constant for me, and my teeth are very happy.

18. Specific to my situation, I continue to make progress every day and will get it all back.

19. Specific to my situation, I am grateful that I am alive and have had great therapists.

Being Properly Thankful

I sent an email to a large distribution list just after Michigan beat Ohio State in football Saturday of Thanksgiving weekend 2021. I needed to make myself feel better. That email was entitled "Being Properly Thankful" and is reproduced for you here:

Fair warning, this email is designed to make you think.

Since I almost died last year, I do not think I had turkey on Thanksgiving or shopped on Black Friday; I feel I am uniquely situated to give you advice on how to be properly thankful:

Take these 5 things into account...

1. Life - I clearly took mine for granted. All I will say is that we know not the hour. Almost dead at 46, yikes! One thing is for

certain, we will all die one day, so be thankful for what you have - you cannot take it with you. I am very thankful to be alive.

2. Health - It is one of the great ironies of my life that I slaved away in the gym daily at work (and ate an apple every day), did not lose any weight, and developed these massive health problems. I earnestly hope you will stay healthy. You should be thankful for your health; use me as an example if it helps.

3. Family - My family has really stepped up in every possible way. I have built up a debt I could never repay, and I would be lost without them. I guess that is the point with family; you do not have to pay back your debts. I am very thankful for my family, as you should be for yours.

4. Friends - a lot of people visited me, took me to lunch, sent me friendly emails, took care of me in other ways, and gave me rides. I am very thankful to have great friends; you all have helped out tremendously.

5. Faith - Without getting too preachy in a wide distribution email, my faith has saved me and continues to do so every day. I am proud to give witness to Jesus Christ and thankful that he is in my life. You should be thankful your God is in your life; it is helpful to know that there is something larger than you are.

So, near this uniquely American holiday, let us be properly thankful.

As a little bit of an update, mostly for those who have not seen me in a while:

It is not all bad, and I continue to make progress every day (I believe, and Kelly believes) I will get back all the way. In fact, yesterday, I tied my shoes for the first time, cut down a Christmas tree, and went to a baseball card show. That said, the season of firsts is ending for me, and the season of getting faster is starting. I can now do most things, albeit slowly. I know I need to get faster at doing things and will focus on that now.

Other good things have happened: I lost 15 pounds, stopped drinking Diet Coke (maybe this caused my stroke, the doctors still do not know*), stopped drinking alcohol (not that I drank that much, I mostly drink water these days), stopped chewing gum (which was a stress-related constant for me), my teeth are much better, am properly thankful, and I think my situation has led one of my sons, Ryan, to find his calling in life. Rest assured, I will keep fighting for every yard with the same type of steely determination you all have known me for. This fight is likely to take years, and with all your help, I will win it. Meliora!

Best,

Kevin

*Fun fact: the cause for about 1/4 of all strokes, including mine, is unknown. For me, a doctor at Johns Hopkins University came the closest to nailing down a cause, and it looks like a blood clot from my leg (or my heart) and traveled to my brain. A freak occurrence that can happen to anyone – unlucky for me. At any rate, what caused my strokes has been and will continue to be, far less important than my recovery.

For you, Meliora is Latin and means "Always Better." It is the alma mater of the school I went to as an undergraduate (The University of Rochester) and, I maintain, perfectly describes what is going on with me.

Church

When talking about thanksgiving, I must talk about Church – because each Mass is like one big group, thanksgiving. We go to Mass every Sunday, every Holy Day of Obligation (in the Catholic Church, there are certain days when Catholics must go to Mass), Ash Wednesday (which is not a holy day of obligation), and Thanksgiving Day (which is also not a holy day of obligation). As for the former, we are into kicking Lent off in style; as for the latter, if you are supposed to give thanks, you better give thanks to the author of all things. We also do not eat meat on Fridays. I figure, if Jesus died for us, not eating meat is the least we can do – I always thought this (and I think the boys will keep doing it). We also say grace every night before dinner – another thing I hope the boys keep up.

Despite all those things, and try as I might, like any good Catholic, I do not feel I make Mass last all week as we should, and feel very guilty about it – and talking has nothing to do with it. All my various Knights of Columbus activities were about making Mass last all week as is our busy contribution schedule; we tithe (and believe God allows us to keep 90%), – we are reminded all week, in the mail, that we are Catholic.

The Knights, seemingly, had events every night. It is a shame those events conflicted with my coaching schedule because the Knights do a lot of great work. I plan to get back to the Knights after the kids have gone. Maybe, I will be an insurance agent. As I mentioned above, the Knights of Columbus is one big insurance company.

I was one of the youngest at most Knights events, and I think I have long thought, there is a certain freedom that comes from being older. I found the group Rosary, which took place on

Mondays, before Council meetings, to be the most useful. There is a certain power that comes from a group of men saying the Rosary, plus you only have to say half the Prayers (the Leader starts each Prayer). The downside of the Rosary was that you must attend the Council meeting – both good and bad. Good because you did get an update on Council events, bad because there was a lot of bloviating (anyone could speak) – which tended to make the meetings last longer. So long, in fact, I wondered, often, if I was the only one with work the next morning. Well, less than 10% of the Council attended the meetings, and I think the length is why. This does not take away from the fact that the Knights do a lot of great work; I will encourage the boys to join (which they can do when they are eighteen) also.

Tithing is an important, though I feel inconsequential, part of our lives. We have always given a lot to charities, as we agree they (mostly) do great work, but I feel my monetary contributions are inadequate. I mean, actions speak louder, and we tend to give out of our surplus. I guess charities share donor lists, because every day, in the mail, we are asked to give money. Daily, we get mail from Catholic organizations asking for money, and we have so many Mass Cards that it is impossible for enough of our acquaintances to die.

A constant theme of my Confessions has been failing to give God thanks for all the great gifts given to me. I have long felt this way, and I still feel this way and will mention this in my next Confession. I plan to talk at my next Confession and have already prepared notes (my next Confession is in a couple of weeks; some things are just too important). I think 'Catholic Guilt' is real. I certainly experience it. I wonder if I will ever feel adequate, no matter how much I do.

Conclusion

The struggle is valuable. It is written in the Bible that "iron sharpeth iron" (Proverbs 27:17); well, there has been a lot of sharpening going on in the Sweeney household. Life is basically a struggle, and without getting too heavy, I mean to convey that there are at least three values in struggle. A lot of ink has been spilled on this theological question. First is the value of proving to yourself that you can do something. Second, there are demonstration effects; that is, as you are struggling you demonstrate to others that your perseverance pays off. Third, there is something unique about a health struggle since we are all likely to face them. It comforts me that my sons will look back on my situation someday, hopefully after I am long gone, and remember how I bucked the trends and fought like hell.

Conclusion

It is appropriate to begin the end by reviewing the two main purposes of this book. First, to stroke survivors and their families, I was (and did) these things. With the proper amount of determination, you can too. You are lucky to be alive, and since strokes are as heterogeneous as the people who have them, maybe your symptoms are less than mine. If so, you are doubly lucky. If not, join the club and prepare for a hard, bumpy ride. I would say an additional two things. First, there is nothing special about me; if I did these things, you can too. Second, do everything your doctors and therapists tell you to do, and then do extra by challenging yourself daily. There is nothing like self-improvement. To my friends and family, I would like to say, I will never stop. I do not care if recovery takes me twenty or more years or if I must write ten books; I pledge to continue to challenge myself every day and do all my doctors and therapists tell me to do. Also, I pledge to continue with the same dry, sarcastic sense of humor you all have known from me.

I begin the conclusion by reviewing my main findings (chapter by chapter), then I talk about our charitable contributions (we have many because we tithe) and the future (college, our serial savings, retirement). I end with a little push to stroke survivors.

In the introduction, we established I have a strong support network; in fact, I cannot imagine going down this road without my wife and kids. To stroke survivors, I would say identify your support network early (and let them know). To friends and family members of stroke survivors, you should prepare to be relied on like never before. Your loved one could have died; many who suffer strokes do. May them being alive be an inspiration to you. To my friends and family, I would simply say thank you. I have built up a debt that I can never repay. I hope I inspire you as much as you inspire me. Know that I am fighting for you and love you.

I felt including the timeline in the first chapter would both be of interest to my family and friends and be insightful for those living through the hell of having a loved one suffer a stroke. The take-home point for my friends and family is that I was incredibly busy at the time of my strokes. I am not sure you all fully appreciated this fact. In the second chapter while stress could certainly have been a factor in my strokes, there is nothing like facing traffic (and a 40-mile commute) when you have to run baseball practice in an hour, given my types of strokes – I do not think so. Nevertheless, I have both reduced the stress in my life and am on two blood-thinning medications (Aspirin and Lipitor) for good measure. For stroke victims and their families, I would say that the dark days will clear up, and then you are in for a battle. Without question, the funniest thing that happened in the first two chapters was me pulling out my tubes and trying to leave the Intensive Care Unit. Classic me. I try to be a good person, but I am not a very good patient.

In the second chapter, What I Was, we established that I was incredibly busy at the time of my strokes and that my inability to talk, Aphasia, affected only certain areas of my life. Where it had an (the biggest) effect (work), that effect was humongous. I blame my Aphasia for losing my job. I would also like to get back to yelling at my kids (sarcasm).

In Chapter Three, I tried to express what I was up to in the months after my strokes. While this has little to do with my Aphasia, which was certainly developing then, it does offer great insight for those about to embark on a post-stroke journey because it tells what you can expect. For my extended friends and family, the chapter offers a blow-by-blow account of what I was going through in which you did not fully participate. Kelly and the boys were there every step of the way. There is no doubt that this was the start of a years-long journey that ends in full recovery. Though there may not seem to be anything funny that happened in this chapter – I would submit scaring my wife and my physical therapist on the stairs is funny. Stairs have always been a nuisance to me to be dealt with as quickly as possible. I think this has to do with having bad knees.

Chapter Four reproduced for you all my missives to Matty's Little League team, and I hope you enjoyed the quotes. The big deal in this chapter was that despite having difficulty talking, I was able to be the head coach of a Little League Baseball team. I am grateful to Upper Loudoun Little League for giving me a chance and very grateful to all the coaches for their help. I would single out my son, Ryan, for his help. Again, for my extended friends and family, this is what my life was like for a decade. I was the head coach for about thirty teams. I moved mountains, as a father should, for my sons. For stroke survivors and their families, the mere fact I was able to do this mere months after my debilitating strokes shows you what is possible. While it appears nothing funny happened in this chapter, watching us play was funny, we were 1-10-1. I would also point out my coaching philosophy did a 180 with this team. I hope my missives displayed that. I went from being a 29-time 'win-at-all-costs' coach to genuinely caring for the kids and if they learned. Little League baseball is meant to be fun, and it only took me a near-death experience to realize that.

Chapter Five, The Land of Falling Trees, detailed some of my biggest accomplishments since the strokes. Oddly, my big accomplishments, or the accomplishments I selected, all seemed to cluster twelve to sixteen months after my strokes. I accomplished these things despite my Aphasia, and they demonstrate what I now value to my friends and family. This chapter is clearly aimed at stroke survivors and their families, and gives you some idea of what to expect and the long road to hoe. It also seems like nothing funny happened in this chapter, but I would submit watching me utterly fail a task the first time I do it is pretty funny.

Chapter Six gives you tremendous insight into what it is like to be me daily. It proves saying I cannot talk is a misnomer, I can – it just takes a tremendous amount of preparation for me to do so. This is what living with my flavor of Aphasia is like for me. My friends and family should be curious about my daily existence, and the chapter gives stroke survivors, and their families, an idea of what to expect moving forward. I certainly hope, in the future, to not have to prepare as much and to sleep through the night. The funniest thing that happened in this chapter was me comparing my current existence to being drunk all the time. Life is really like that for me, except there is no pleasure and no hangover… a shame because I know some great cures for hangovers.

Finally, in Chapter Seven, I end on a hopeful note. There is no question my sons have learned tremendous life-long lessons from my struggles and the actions of Kelly. Everybody ought to keep a gratuity journal, and it is helpful to believe something out there is bigger than you. For my friends and family, I show what I value these days (if anyone has any additions, they should let me know).

For stroke survivors and their families, chapter seven demonstrates that you may not have to look hard for silver linings to your predicament. There is nothing funny about these lessons and, as I said, everyone should keep a gratuity journal; there is good, scientific, evidence that doing so positively affects your brain.

I will conclude this section by saying I will not stay like this forever; in fact, I am learning and growing every day. My prognosis is to fully recover, a process that will take years. The doctors say my age and determination will win the day, and the fact that I had no pre-existing conditions bodes well for me. Writing this book was part of my therapy. Many people my age search for meaning in their life. Kelly and I know our purpose in life and will not have a midlife crisis. We are to battle, and victory will be glorious.

Charitable Contributions

It is fitting for me to end with charitable contributions, both because it is a big part of our life, and we think everybody should tithe. Admittedly, this has little to do with my inability to talk. However, I blame my current employment situation on my Aphasia, which will affect my income and close one important door to me. In this section, I detail our charitable contributions. As an example, for all readers. Most importantly, we contribute a great deal to charity; as I pointed out above, we tithe. That is, tithe.

Weekly, we donate to Church in the Sunday collection basket. We put a lot of money in the basket (the former Pastor published, in the bulletin, the anonymous contributions he got, and our dollar value was the near the top). This is the most scalable of our donations, and I have already let the current Pastor know that our weekly contribution will fluctuate and, probably, decrease.

I contributed to the Combined Federal Campaign (CFC). The CFC is a federal giving campaign where Federal Employees can select from a list of charities (hundreds of them) and have money taken directly out of their paycheck to go to those charities. We gave our money to Catholic Charities of Arlington and KOVAR, a Knights of Columbus Charity that helps people in Virginia with intellectual disabilities. I had this money taken out of my paycheck, biweekly.

Monthly, we have two charitable donations. First, we contribute to Food for the Poor. Food for the Poor Food began in 1982 in Jamaica. Today, this Christian Ministry serves the poor in 17 countries throughout the Caribbean and Latin America. They provide things like food, housing, healthcare, education, fresh water, emergency relief, and micro-enterprise solutions. We started donating when a very effective Missionary came to our Parish about a decade ago. At the time, we were looking for a monthly charity, and this one seemed to fit the bill. Clearly, they give out our contact information, because we get lots of mail from them and other charitable organizations. We could stop donating, but I do not want to as I plan to use this with St. Peter at the gates of heaven. We also 'contribute' monthly with our Knights of Columbus insurance premiums. As I mentioned above, the Knights are, basically, an insurance company, and both Kelly and I have life insurance through them. The insurance is costly, but the premiums are used to support a host of Knights Charities. Not many Knights, about 10%, are 'insurance members.' This monthly contribution is not, at all, scalable.

Monthly, we also donate food to our Parish. The Parish Knights of Columbus collect the food and drop it off a local food pantry. The Parish has donated tons of food over time, and I am proud to say we contributed a large share to that. But my newfound freedom should enable me to help with either boxing up, or delivering, the food.

Like a lot of people, we had some end-of-year contributions that we made, looking for tax breaks. We used to gift each other for Christmas contributions to Project Rachel and Gabriel Project. Both are Diocese of Arlington Charities that support right-to-life campaigns. Gabriel Project supports crisis pregnancies including buying diapers and other items, transportation to doctors visits, and donations of furniture, clothes and toys. Project Rachel provides post-abortion counseling services to both women and men. Finally, both Kelly and I went to two schools and both University level and Department level opportunities to contribute annually – which we tended to do, but probably, will not do anymore.

You round this out with a bevy of random contributions (such as free will offerings at Parish pancake breakfasts) you get a well-rounded charitable giving picture. I thought it appropriate to mention all this in conclusion, though it has little to do with my inability to talk (at least directly) because it is/was a big part of our lives, and we believe, firmly, the world would be a better place if all people were more charitable. So, if we can inspire one person, or family, to do so, we have done our job.

Retirement

In a very real sense, Kelly and I are perfect for each other... we are both cheap. We tend not to spend money on what most other people spend money on, such as music, movies/going out, and clothes. We will never get leather seats for our cars, if power windows were an option we would, certainly, crank ours. The strokes have not changed my worldview, I am still a saver. Because of this, thank God, we have a great deal of money saved for retirement already. We are ahead of the game and only in our middle 40s. In this section, I will share about our very cool, plan for retirement. None of this has to do with my inability to talk and instead points to a future that is happy and bright, after we do a tremendous amount of work.

We have always planned to retire to Cooperstown, New York. There is a lake there that Kelly really likes, and the town is nice, and, of course, the Baseball Hall of Fame is there. I am no longer sure we will be right on the lake, but I still intend to volunteer at the Hall of Fame and die in front of Babe Ruth's locker – which is there (if you have not been to the Baseball Hall of Fame, I will encourage you to go). Kelly wants a second place to live near the boys and away from the upstate New York winters, and I do not care now, though I want to live near the boys too. Nevertheless, she will get whatever she wants; no doubt she deserves it. Our plans have not changed because of my condition and will not.

The Grand Conclusion

In terms of the faraway future, there are things I know, things I think, and things I am unsure of. That is how I organize this grand conclusion. One thing is certain, my list of maladies, including lacking verbal communication, is temporary.

I know that Matty will age out of Little League this Spring, and I will not coach anymore (I do wonder what I will do with all the stuff I have accumulated. I am trying to give some of it away now. Kelly plans a garage sale). I plan to Umpire when I can. I know Ryan will graduate high school and go to college in 2023. Timmy will follow him in 2025 and Matty in 2028. I am certain that when we move out of this house, it will be a chore. There is no way around it, and we will have a lifetime of accumulated stuff.

I also know I will never stop fighting. Never. Neither should you. My prognosis is one of full recovery (my doctors think my age, determination, and the fact I had no pre-existing conditions all bode well for me), and I intend to get there. I do not care if it takes twenty years or if I must write ten books. If you had a stroke, you should fight hard and never give up. Challenge yourself daily. I also know my friends and family will continue to support me. They will hardly be surprised by my determination. Lastly, I know Kelly and I will be together forever. Forever. We are high school sweethearts and have been trying for eighty years. 1992, so we have a chance, 2072.

I think Ryan will play baseball at a Division III college and will major in kinesiology, and become a physical therapist. He, they all, will be great fathers (I suppose I am certain). I think Timmy will run at a Division 1 school and become an Engineer. He is a talented enough runner, if he stays healthy, that he can run at that level, and he has the mind of an engineer. I think Matty will go into Information Technology (IT), certainly, his love for screens is such that he should roll this into a career. I also think the boys will say grace before dinner, be life-long churchgoers, and coach baseball. I think Kelly and I have set a strong example for them, and there is no question they have learned some essential lessons from this ordeal.

I am not sure the boys, or any of you, will keep a gratuity journal. It is a lot of work. Try putting it on your bedstand and filling it in every night right before you go to bed. I am also not certain we have saved enough money for retirement. I suppose this feeling is familiar to all who are reading this book. Most people feel they have not saved enough for retirement. It is a little like a bottomless pit. I am not certain how long our cars will last. We put a lot of miles on them for years, less so now. But, with Ryan driving, and Timmy hot on his heels, there is little doubt we will need another car eventually and will burn through the ones we have more quickly. I am also not certain how long our appliances will last. We are replacing some now and have a plan to replace the rest.

Finally, I am not at all certain of how long I will have to fight. I am prepared for a years-long battle, and you should be too.

Dr. Kevin Sweeney was the Senior Advisor for the Directorate of Strategic and Operational Planning (DSOP) at the National Counterterrorism Center (NCTC) at the Office of the Director of National Intelligence (ODNI). Prior to that, he was a Group Chief in DSOP. Previously was the Group Chief for Data, Tools, and Methods inside the Studies and Evaluations Division in ODNI Systems and Resource Analysis (SRA). Dr. Sweeney worked at ODNI from 2010 to 2022. He was promoted to the Senior National Intelligence Service in 2017. Beginning his government service in 2004, he spent 6 years at the Joint Warfare Analysis Center (JWAC) in Dahlgren, VA. Dr. Sweeney received his Ph.D. in Political Science from The Ohio State University in 2004, and a Bachelor's degree in Political Science and History from the University of Rochester in 1996. He is a, many times over, published author. Dr. Sweeney was born and raised in Levittown, NY, and is married to the former Ms. Kelly Lynn Byrnes of Oceanside, NY. They reside in Purcellville, Virginia, with their sons Ryan, Timothy, and Matthew.

REFERENCES

The 25 biggest college football stadiums in the country |
    NCAA.com, accessed 1 February 2022.

Berra, Yogi Various dates. Quotes from
    https://quotecatalog.com/communicator/ted-williams/
    accessed in the fall and summer of 2021

Brown, Joshua and Kolton Wong. 2017, "How Gratitude
    Changes You and Your Brain," accessed online (January 23,
    2023):
    https://greatergood.berkeley.edu/article/item/how_gratitude_
    changes_you_and_your_brain

Coll, Steven. *Directorate S: The C.I.A. and America's Secret
    Wars in Afghanistan and Pakistan.* Penguin Press, 2018.

Flanagan, Thomas. *The Year of the French.* Henry Holt and
    Company, Inc. 1979.

Fritz, Paul, and Kevin Sweeney. 2004e "The (De)limitations of
    Balance of Power Theory." *International Interactions*
    30(4):285-308.

Gortzak, Yoav, Yoram Haftel, and Kevin Sweeney. 2005a. "Offense-Defense Theory: An Empirical Assessment." Journal of Conflict Resolution 49(1):67-89.

Graves, Robert. *Goodbye to All That.* Penguin Modern Classics, 2000.

Hersh, Seymour M. *Chain of Command: The Road from 9/11 to Abu Ghraib.* Harper, 2004.

Hillenbrand, Laura. *Unbroken: An Olympian's Journey from Airman to Castaway to Captive.* Delacorte Press, 2014.

Lacey, Robert. *Inside the Kingdom: Kings, Clerics, Modernists, Terrorists, and the Struggle for Saudi Arabia.* Penguin Books, 2009.

Lustick, Ian S. *Trapped in the War on Terror.* University of Pennsylvania Press, 2006.

McDonald, Patrick and Kevin Sweeney. 2007. "The Achilles' Heel of Liberal IR Theory? Globalization and Conflict in the Pre World War One Era. *World Politics* 59(3): 370-403.

Paige, Satchel Various dates. Quotes from https://quotecatalog.com/communicator/ted-williams/ accessed in the fall and summer of 2021

Plaut, David. 1992. Baseball Wit and Wisdom. The Running Press.

Shanker, Thom and David S. Cloud. February 7, 2007. "Military Wants More Civilians to Help in Iraq." New York Times

Sookhdeo, Patrick. *Unmasking the Islamic State: Revealing Their Motivation, Theology, and End Time Predictions.* Isaac Publishing, 2015.

Sweeney, Kevin. 2003. "The Severity of Interstate Disputes: Are Dyadic Capability Preponderances Really More Pacific?" *Journal of Conflict Resolution* 74(6):728-50.

Sweeney, Kevin. 2005c. "The Assessment of Non-Physical Human Factors in the Context of the Naval Capability Evolution Process." *International Council on Systems Engineering Insight* 8(1): 23.

Sweeney, Kevin. 2004 a-c. "Heteroskedasticity," "Regression Coefficient," "Regression Toward the Mean," in *The Encyclopedia of Social Science Research Methods*, Michael

Lewis-Beck, Alan Bryman, and Tim Futing Liao eds. Thousand Oaks, California: Sage.

Sweeney, Kevin and Brock Edwards. 2012. "The Intelligence Community's Global Posture." *Studies in Intelligence*

Sweeney, Kevin, and Paul Fritz. 2004d. "Jumping on the Bandwagon: An Interest Based Explanation for Great Power Alliances," *Journal of Politics* 66(2):428-49.

Sweeney, Kevin and Omar M.G. Khesk. 2005b. "The Similarity of States: Using S to Compute Dyadic Interest Similarity." *Conflict Management and Peace Science*

Williams, Ted. Various dates. Quotes from https://quotecatalog.com/communicator/ted-williams/ accessed in the fall and summer of 2021.

Wright, Lawrence. *The Looming Tower: Al-Qaeda and the Road to 9/11.* Vintage Books, 2007.

INDEX

A

Aaron Junk, 128, 136, 137
Abdul Dostum, 81
Abdullah Abdullah, 80
Ability Fitness, 77
Abraham Lincoln
(Washington Nationals
Mascot), 155
Afghanistan, 79-87
Atrial Fibrillation (Afib), 22
African American History
Museum, 166
Ahmed Shah Massoud, 80,
84
Ahmed Wali, 85
Al Arbour, 45
Al Kaline, 158
Alabama (University of), 50
Alphonse Niedermeyer, 31,
114-115
Al-Qaeda, 84
Altar Server, 187, 188
'America the Beautiful', 154
American Journal of Politics,
33
American League, 155
American League Most
Valuable Player Award, 53
Americana, 157, 186

Americans with Disabilities
Act, 179
Amrullah Salah, 82
Anbar Province, 17
Andy Trice, 167
Angelica Joy Neidermeyer,
114
Ann Arbor, MI 50
Anne Quinn, x
Aparma Iyer, viii, 66
Aphasia, i, iv, xii, 60, 172,
176, 181, 209, 210, 212
Ash Wednesday, 205
Ashaf Kayani, 81
Asprin, 209
Augustus Poisson, 32

B

Babe Ruth, v, 112, 215
Baltimore, MD 153, 158, 160
Baltimore Aquarium, 153,
166
Baltimore's Inner Harbor,
153
Baltimore Oriole (Mascot),
155
Baltimore Orioles, 153, 155
Baseball, v, 27-29, 41, 42,
44-45, 57, 61, 87, 91-143,

154-156, 163, 185, 186, 195, 209, 216

Baseball caps (Hats), 63

Baseball Card Collecting, 41, 43, 51-56, 60, 156, 157

Baseball card show, 61, 157-158, 159, 203

Baseball fields, 143, 190

Baseball Hall of Fame, 45, 107, 215

Baseballs, 28

Baseeball gloves, 28

Basketball, v, 14, 27, 28, 42, 48, 49, 51, 91, 164-165

Batman, 185

Batting gloves, 28

Batting helmets, 28

Benoit Hogue, 57

Bible, 207

Big East Conference, 49

Bill Dickey, 118

Bill Torrey, 45

Bill Veeck, 119, 125

Billy Smith, 45

Bioness Integrated Therapy System (BITS), 78

Bishop of Arlington, 176

BJ Phillips, 104

Black Friday, 202

Blarney Stone, ii, iii

Blue Ridge Middle School Baseball Team, 92

Bob Villatore, 47

Bookmarketers, x

Bowie Kuhn, 123

Bowman, 52, 53

Branch Rickey, 120

Brock Edwards, 33

Brooklyn Dodgers, 44, 120, 137

Brushing your teeth, ii

Bryant-Denny Stadium, 50

Buffalo Sabers, 57

Business casual, 179

Butch Goring, 45

Buttoning jeans, iii

C

Camden Yards, 153, 155

Carl Yastrzemski, 158

Casey White, x

CAT scan, 15, 16, 19, 21

Catholic, 18, 36, 76, 201, 205, 206

Catholic Charities of Arlington, 213

Catholic Guilt, 206

CCD (Confraternity of Christian Doctorine), 187, 190

Central Loudoun Little League (CLLL), 108, 116, 122, 124, 134

Cerebral aneurism, 21, 59

Chairman of the Joint Chiefs of Staff, 82, 177

Channel 9 (NY), 42, 44

Charles Sweeney, 56, 58-59

Chris Byrnes, vi

Chris Matthew, x

Chris Mullin, 49

Chris Thompson, 92, 97, 99-100, 102, 105, 110, 112, 114, 118, 121, 122, 125, 126, 127, 129, 130, 133, 134, 141, 142
Chris Wood, 82, 84
Christine Ristano, ix, 90
Christmas, 40, 54, 75, 76, 87, 147, 148, 158, 159, 160, 161, 162, 214
Christmas Card, 159
Christmas Lights, 160
Christmas List, 161
Christmas Tree, 61, 158, 159, 203
Cleaning my glasses, iii
Coach, iv, v, viii, x, xi, 24, 27-29, 40, 45, 49, 63, 91-143, 165, 180, 181, 183, 184, 186, 191, 197, 205, 210, 216
Coach Kevin, 91-143
Cody and Cooper Sweeney, vi
Cody ICU nurse, viii
Cofer Black, 80
College Football Preview Magazine, 156
College Station, Texas, 50
Columbia University, 49
Columbus, Ohio, 50, 59
Combined Federal Campaign, 213
Confession, 206
Connor and Hannah Byrnes, vi
Cooperstown, NY, 215
COSTCO, 189

COVID, 15, 18, 25, 65, 66, 68, 95, 98, 117, 144, 145, 179

D

Daily Missal, 189
Dale Weaver, ix
Damon Stevens, vi, 26, 166
Dan Marino, 48, 54
Darrell Green, 55
Dave Winfield, 43
David Dinkins, 30, 114
David Petraeus, 82
David Sedney, 84
Denis Potvin, 45

Diet Coke, 61, 182, 204
Diocese of Arlington, 214
Directorate of Strategic and Operational Planning, vi, 27, 144-149, 166-168, 176-178, 218
Disney, 156-157
District All Stars, 28, 91, 94
Division Avenue High School, 47
Division I, 216
Division III, 218
Dizzy Dean, 128
Do not call list, 171
Doing ' the book', 164-165
Doing laundry, 40, 177
Don Mattingly, 43, 44, 54
Donald Rumsfeld (Rumsfeldian), 32, 80, 85, 86, 88-89

Donruss, 51, 52, 54
Donut, 27
Do-re-me, 174, 175
Doris Kearns Godwin, 134
Douglas Lute, 82, 84
Downstate New York, 48
Dr. Ashiny, viii
Dr. Choudhary, viii
Dr. Cindy Lee, viii, 16

Dr. Gaddipati, viii
Dr. Geloo, ix, 71
Dr. Jill Bode Taylor, 178
Dr. Meagan Cooper, viii
Dr. Mei Firestone, ix, 72,
Dr. Nadim, ix
Dr. Rafeal Llinas, ix, 71, 160
Dr. Ramesh, viii
Dr. Rana, viii
Dr. Seth Tuwiner, ix, 72
Dr. Shetal Patel, ix
Drazen Petrovich, 42
Driving, i, iv, 41, 52, 59-60,
147, 149, 190, 191, 217
Dwight D. Eisenhower, 137
Dwight Gooden, 56

E

Easter Sunday, 182
Ed Scott, 46
Edmonton Oilers, 45
Ehsan ul-Haq, 81
Elevate (elevateapp.com), 88,
149-150
elevenwarriors.com, 48

Elisabeth Graham, ix, 70, 73,
74, 87, 88, 175
Eminey Gullmaz, x
Encompass Health, viii, 23,
61-70, 72, 73, 89, 151, 180,
184, 202
Encyclopedia of Social
Science Research Methods,
31
Engineer Arif, 80
Eric Dickerson, 55
ESPN, 92
evite.com, 167
Executive Core
Qualifications, 178
Ezekiel Elliot, 191

F

Facebook, 163
Fairfax County Public
Schools (Virginia), vi
Fantasy Football, 190
Father Gould, x, 18
Father Heisler, x
Fleer, 51, 52, 54
Florida, vii, 156
fMRI scanner, 198, 199
Food for the Poor, 213
Football, xi, 42, 47-51, 65,
75, 156, 185, 190, 202
Football Card Collecting, 52,
54, 55, 176
Foreign Affairs, 35, 80
Formula One Racing, 65

Franklin Park 133, 135, 136, 137, 138
Freakonomics, 176

G

Gabe Paul, 139
Gabriel Project, 214
Gala apples, 183, 189
Gamechanger, 94
George Tenet, 82
George W. Bush, 82
Georgetown University, 49
Gerard Skinner, viii
Gilligan's Island, 186
God, 76, 107, 123, 134, 160, 196, 203, 205, 206, 215
God-Given, 196
Grace, 180, 205, 216
Gratuity journal, 198, 200, 211, 212, 217
Greg Hodges, 112, 118, 121, 131-135, 142
Gregg Burgess, ix, 167
Group Chief, 25, 177, 218
Gul Agha Sherzai, 82

H

Halloween, 71
Hamid Karzai, 81
Hamilton Elementary School 102, 105, 119, 120
Happy Birthday, 175
Hapsburg Empire, 202
Hard Rock Cafe, 153
Hardcore History, 176

Harvard, 30
Haske Field (Purcellville, VA), 96, 98, 100, 102, 104, 106, 109, 110, 112, 114, 116, 118, 119, 121, 124, 125, 126, 129, 130, 133, 134, 137, 138, 139
Heart monitor, ix, 23, 70, 71, 75, 78
Heather (at INOVA), 76
Heavy balls, 27
Helen Parker, ix, 77, 90, 201
Helicopter, i, 17
Hempstead Turnpike, 46
Heparin, 21
Hepatitis, 56
Herb Caen, 121
Herbert Weisberg, 33
Hezbollah, 87
Hilary Clinton, 81
Hockey, 51, 55
Hockey cards, 55
Hofstra University, 46
Holy Day of Obligation, 76, 205
Holy Orders, 18
Holy Trinity Council, Knights of Columbus 7812, 37
Honus Wagner, 137
Hospital Bed, 69, 70-72, 151
Hotel, 160, 161
Huber Field (Leesburg, VA), 116

I

Ian Lustick, 79
Ibraham Haqqani, 81
Intensive Care Unit (ICU), i, viii, 15, 16, 22, 58, 59, 195, 209
Independence Day, 149
India, 87
Indiana University, 49
Cleveland Indians, 59, 125
INOVA Cornwall, i, viii, 14
INOVA Fairfax, viii, 17
INOVA Loudoun, i, viii, 15, 76-78, 87
Insurance Agent (Knights of Columbus), 37, 205
Interaction effect, 31
Interactive Metronome (IM), 74
International Council on Systems Engineering Insight Journal, 32
International Interactions, 31
International Security, 35
Interview Panels, 26
iPad, 74
Iraq, 17, 80, 85, 86

J

Jackie (at INOVA), 76
Jacques Barzun, 107
Jamaica, 63, 213
James Marsh, ix, 92, 97, 100, 103, 105, 109, 132, 135, 138, 1398, 142

Jamie Sweeney, vi
Janet Box-Steffensmeier, x, 33
Jason Bartolomei, x, 28, 75
Jay's Wintery Mix, 163
Jesus Christ, 145, 203, 205
Jim Jones, 81
Jim McMahon, 54
Joe DiMaggio, 114, 124
Joe Montana, 55
John Byrnes, vii, x, 58, 191
John Brennan, 80
John Elway, 55
John Sterling, 44
Johns Hopkins University, ii, ix, 19, 71, 160, 204
Joint Warfare Analysis Center (JWAC), 32, 218
Journal of Conflict Resolution, 30
Journal of Politics, 31

K

Kalman Filters, 163
Kansas City Royals, 128
Karl Eikenberry, 81
Kashmir, 87
Kathleen Sweeney, 36, 51, 56, 58-59, 159
Kelly Sweeney, iv-vii, x, 13, 15-19, 21-23, 24, 26, 35, 40, 41, 54, 58, 61, 63-65, 69, 73, 75, 76, 87-89, 93, 95, 99, 101, 102, 109, 110, 116, 147,

148, 151-153, 156-3, 172,
173, 175-180, 183, 184, 186-
191, 194, 196, 197, 200, 203,
210, 211-216, 218
Kelly Gaffney, ix
Kelly Moran, ix, 78, 90
Ken O'Brien, 48
Kerry Rice, ix, 140
Kim Smith, x, 179
Kinesiology, 216
Knights of Columbus K of
C), x, 35-38, 205, 206, 213,
214
KOVAR, 213
Kris Wershinsky, ix
Krista, ix, 73
Kulika Frazier, vi, 27
Kyle Field (College Station,
TX), 50

L

Labor Day, 104
LaGuardia Airport, 30, 114
Laser Surgery, iii
Last Rites, 13, 18
Latin America, 213
Laura Hillenbrand, 79
Laura Serine, ix, 76, 78, 79,
87, 90, 191
Laurel, ix, 73, 90
Lawrence Ritter, 138
Lawrence Taylor, 54
Lector, 187, 189
Lector workbook, 187

Leesburg, VA, 14, 73, 77,
116, 117, 122, 123, 124
Lefty O'Doul, 111
Lent, 182, 205
Leo Durocher, 101
Leon Panetta, 82
Lester Holt, 181
Levittown, NY, 47, 57, 218
Lewis Hamilton, 65
Lipitor, 21, 209
Little League, viii, ix, x, 24,
29, 92, 93, 109. 100, 126,
141, 143, 155, 197, 210, 211,
215
, 29, 95, 155
Little League Baseball, viii,
ix, 24, 28, 92, 109, 125, 139,
140, 154, 197, 210, 211, 216
Little League World Series,
108
Liz Byrnes, vi
Los Angles (and Brooklyn)
Dodgers, 44, 120, 137
Lou Carnesecca, 49
Loudoun Couty Fair, 39
Loudoun County Parks and
Recreation, 131
Loudoun Valley High
School, v, 92, 174
Lowell Cohn, 112
Louisiana State University
(LSU), 50
lumosity.com, 74, 149

M

Macy's, 75

Madison Square Garden Network, 42

Mahmud Ahmed, 80

Major League Baseball Extra Innings, 13

Mardi Gras, 148

Margie Comford, ix, 67, 76, 87-90, 149, 150, 175, 187

Maria Hurst, viii, 68, 70, 73,

Marines, 17

Mario Valenti, ix, 98, 140

Mark Jackson, 49

Mary had a Little Lamb, 175

Mass, 38, 75, 76, 187, 189, 190, 205,

Mass Cards, 206

Matthew James Arroyo, 41, 56-7, 195

Matty Sweeney, v, viii, 13, 29, 35, 76, 91-93, 117, 140, 154, 157, 164, 180, 183, 185, 188, 191, 197, 201, 210, 216, 218

Megan (PT assistant), 72, 90, 151, 152

Meghan Powell, ix, 90

Melatonin, 181

Meliora, 61, 204

Michael Flynn, 81

Michael J. McGivney, 36,

Michael Kaye, 44

Michele Flournoy, 84

Michelle Villarreal, viii, 67-68

Michigan Stadium, 50

Mickey Mantle, 53

Middle School Baseball Team, 28, 29, 92

Middle Schoolers Acting for Christ: Prayer Action Charity (MAC-PAC), 191

Mike Bossy, 45, 55

Mike D'Andrea, 81

Mike Hayden, 81

Mike Mullen, 82

Mountain View Elementary School, 110, 126, 127, 129

the Lawn, 190

MRI, 15, 16, 19, 21

N

Nancy Neidermeyer, 114

NASCET, 20

Nassau Coliseum, Uniondale, NY, 46

National Aquarium, 153

National Counterterrorism Center vi, 25, 30, 218

National League, 155

National Weather Service, 163

Washington Nationals, 154-155

Nativity Set, 160, 162

NATO, 31, 82, 181

NBC, 47

NBC Nightly News, 181, 185

NCAA.com, 50

Nebraska University, 48

Neural sensitivity, 198

Neuroplasticity, 74, 88
New Jersey Nets, 42,
New Year's Day, 76
New Year's Resolution, iii
New Year's Ball Drop, 76
New York, vii, 21, 43, 44, 47-8, 57, 59, 176, 215
New York Giants (Football), 42
New York Islanders, 42, 45-46, 57, 176, 201
New York Jets, 42, 46 - 48, 54, 176, 201
New York Knicks, 42
New York Mets, 42, 44, 47, 57
New York Rangers, 42, 57
New York Times, 17, 32, 35, 176
New York Yankees, i, 13, 41-5, 51, 59, 118, 134, 139, 154, 155, 176, 180, 201
New Yorkers, 42
Neyland Stadium, Knoxville, TN, 50
NFL Red Zone, 190, 191
NHL Center Ice, 45
Nick Denizli, viii, 67-68, 176
Nolan Ryan, 53
Non-Fluent Aphasia, iv, 172, 176, 181
Nor Easter, 163
Northern Virginia, i, 39, 59, 62, 163

Nurses Evelyn, Kailyn, Angie, Molly, Courtney, and Crystal, viii

O

Occupational Therapist, iv, ix, 21, 22, 173
Occupational Therapy (OT), viii, 67, 68, 69, 72, 73, 76, 78, 89, 146
Oceanside, NY 218
ODNI Systems and Resource Analysis (SRA), 218
Offense-Defense Theory, 31
Office of Personnel Management, 24, 178
Office of the Director of National Intelligence (ODNI), vi, 82, 147, 218
Ohio Stadium, Columbus, OH 50
Ohio State Buckeyes, 42, 48, 191, 201
Ohio State University (OSU), ix, 32-33, 48, 49, 50, 51, 58, 176, 180, 185, 202, 218
Oklahoma Football, 48
Olympics, 185
Omar Khesk, 32
O-Pee-Chee, 55
Osama Bin Laden, 80, 83, 84, 86

P

Pakistan, 79-81, 83, 84, 86, 87

Pancreatic Cancer, 167
Parkinson's Disease, 195
Pasadena, California, 76
Pastor, 18, 212, 213
Pat LaFontaine, 46, 56, 57
Pat McDonald, x, 32
Pat Sweeney, vi, 58, 59
Patellar Tendon, 14
Patent Foramen Ovale (PFO), ii, 23, 71
Patrick Flatley, 46
Patrick Sookhdeo, 79
Paul Fritz, 31
Paul Gallico, 127
Paul McGuire, 47
Paul Thomson, x
President's Daily Brief (PDB), 25
Peanut M and Ms, 156
Pedometer challenge, 147
Penn State University, 50
Pepsi, 46
Pete Rose, 53
Peter Chiarelli, 17
Peter Lavoy, 82
PEWMA model, 32
Phil Rizzuto, 43, 53
Philip Roth, 130
Physical Therapist, ix, 22, 151, 201, 210, 216,
Physical Therapy, viii, 16, 66, 68, 69, 72, 73, 76, 89, 146, 151, 152, 182, 199, 201, 208, 214
Physician's Assistants Karen, Jen, and Susan, viii

Pittsburgh Pirates, 180
Playing the Keyboard, 88
Port Authority Police Officers, 30, 114
Porter Goss, 81
Prayers, x, 181, 189, 206
Prefrontal cortex, 198, 199
President Barack Obama, 86
Presidents Day, 166
Priest, 188, 201
Project Rachel, 214
Proverbs, 207
Purcellville, v, 159, 218
Putting on a band-aid, iii

R

Randall Schweller, 33
Reavis Field (Leesburg, VA), 124
Red Smith, 115
Referee, 165
Reggie White, 55
Retirement, 6, 24, 25, 208, 214-215, 217
Revise and Resubmit, 34
Richard Cheney, 83
Richard Blee, 80, 83
Richard Holbrooke, 81, 84, 85
Ricky Parker, ix, 70, 73, 74, 152
Rip Van Winkle, 123
River Bandits (ULLL), 92 - 94 103, 105, 114, 134, 139, 141

Robert Graves, 79
Robert Lacey, 79
Roger Angell, 118
Ronnie Lott, 55
Rosary, 39, 205-206
Rose Bowl, 76, 162, 180
Row, Row, Row Your Boat, 175
Roy Campanella, 137
Russ Grimm, 55
Russia, 181
Rusty, 44, 58
Ryan Cusack, ix, 76, 77, 201
Ryan Sweeney, v, x, 13, 14, 27-29, 35, 40, 41, 42, 57, 59, 61, 91-94, 97, 99-102, 105, 111, 135, 142, 154, 155-157, 160-162, 183, 187, 188, 191, 197, 201, 204, 210, 216, 217, 218

S

Sacrament, 18
Saint John Paul the Second, 194
San Francisco, 47, 121
San Francisco Giants, 180
Sandy Koufax, 125
Satchel Paige, 108, 109, 114, 117, 119, 122, 123, 126, 128, 129, 131, 134, 136, 139
Schottenstein Center, 51
Score, 52, 54,

Scott Jenkins Field (Hamilton, VA), 96, 102-104, 106-108, 110, 112, 116, 118, 119, 121-124, 126-128, 130-132, 135-138, 141, 142
Scranton/Wilkes-Barre Railriders, 176
Seattle Mariners, 43, 51
Secretary of Defense, 177
Senior Advisor, 25, 26, 218
Senior Executive, 25, 88, 167, 178
September 11th, 30, 114
Serena Lambert, 166
Seroquel, 21
Service Academies, 48
Seymour Hersh, 79
Shamrock, 19
Shaquille O'Neal, 31
Shaving, 41, 71, 175, 182, 186
Sherry Barnes, 178
Shoeless Joe, 132
Shot in the Stomach, 66
Shoveling snow, 151,162-163, 171
Showering, vii, 25, 66-68, 73, 88, 160, 172, 175-176, 183, 186
Shutterfly, 159
Singing in a Choir, 88, 189
Sirach, vi
Sirus XM Radio, 150
skill*effort, 196
Senior National Intelligence Service (SNIS), 24-25, 178

snore, 152
Snow Blower, 162
Solemnity of Mary, 76
Speech Therapist, ix, 21, 22,
67, 70, 89, 149, 175, 187
Speech Therapy, viii, 22, 67,
73, 74, 86-89, 175
Speech-Language and
Literacy Center, 74
Spencer Neilson, viii, ix
Spinal tap, 15
Sports Channel, 42
Spring Break, 153
St. Augustine, 189
St. Bernard's Roman
Catholic Church, 57
St. Francis de Sales Roman
Catholic Parish, v, x, 37-39,
212, 214
St. John Arena (Columbus,
OH), 51
St. John's University
Basketball, 48-49
St. Patrick's Day, 148
St. Peter, 213
St. Thomas Aquinas, 201
Stanley Cup, 45, 46
Stanley McCrystal, 82
Steve Busby, 128
Steve Heidorn, 167
Steve Young, 55
Steve Yzerman, 55
Steven Coll, 79
Studies in Intelligence, 33
Super Bowl, 46
Super Mommy, 194, 196

Susan Grant, ix
Swallow test, 22, 68
Sweeney Family, v,76, 94,
139, 197, 207

T

Take me out to the Ball
Game, 154, 174, 175
Taking in the garbage cans,
178
Taking off a suit, 25, 179,
180
Taliban, 84 - 86
Tallulah Bankhead, 136
Team Snap, 93, 96, 98, 99,
101, 104, 105, 109, 110, 112,
116, 133, 135
Ted Williams, 107, 111, 113,
117, 119, 121, 123, 124, 126,
129, 131, 133, 135, 195
Tee Ball, 28, 91
TEE test, 22, 23
Tees, 27
Tennis balls, 27
Terry McLaren, 191
Texas A&M University, 50
Text, 40-41
thank you notes, 200
Thanksgiving, 75, 157, 158,
202, 205
The ABC Song, 175
The Beatles, 150
The Washington Post, 35
Thomas Flanagan, 79
Tied my shoes, 61, 164, 203

Tiger Stadium (Batton Rouge, LA), 50
Timmy Sweeney, v, 13, 17, 27, 29, 38, 54, 57, 76, 91, 154, 162, 183, 185, 188, 190, 191, 192, 197, 216-218
Tithing, 206
Topps, 51-53, 55, 158
tPA, i, 15
Traumatic Brain Injuries, 63
Travel Baseball, 28, 186
Tree Farm, 158, 159
Trice Bowl, 166, 167
tropicaltibits.com, 163
TSA, 156
Twin Towers, 30, 114
Tying my shoes, 61, 151, 164, 203
Typing, iii, 78

U

Ukraine, 181
Umpire, 29, 98, 103
United States, iii, 36, 132, 181, 185
United States Capitol, 75
United States Government, 24, 128
United States Supreme Court, 147
University of Michigan, 50, 108, 200, 202
University of Rochester, 61, 204, 218
University of Tennessee, 50

Upper Deck, 52
Upper Loudoun Little League (ULLL), ix, 92, 96, 101, 109, 116, 118, 132, 134, 140, 210
Upstate New York, 47, 59, 215
US Airways, 30, 114
USA Today, 35

V

Valdimir Putin, 181
Villanova University, 50

W

W.P. Kinsella, 132
Washington DC, 75
Wayne Gretzky, 45, 55
Wearing a belt, 179
Wearing a shirt, 180
Wearing a suit, 25, 179, 180
Wearing a tee-shirt, 179
Wearing a tie, 179
Wearing boots, 164
Wearing glasses, iii, iv,
Wearing shoes, 61, 151, 164, 179, 187, 188, 192, 203
Wearing socks, viii, 63, 67, 105, 192
Wearing underwear, 63, 179
Wedding Vows, 196
Weed whacking the lawn, 190
Wendy Chamberlin, 81
Wesley Walker, 48
Wesley Wood, x

White House Situation
Room, 84
Wiffleball, 27
William Patchak, x
William Shakespeare, 136
Williamsport, PA, 92
Willie Mays, 136
Winchester, VA 157
Winter sports, 185
World Politics, 33
World Series, 44, 180
World War One, 33
WPIX 11, 43
Wrapped Christmas Presents,
161
"Wonderland", 47

Y

Yankee Stadium, 106, 180
YES, 44
Yoav Gortzak, 31
Yogi Berra, 43, 47, 53, 101,
102, 106, 109, 111, 112, 116,
118, 119, 120, 122, 125, 128,
130, 132, 134
Yoram Haftel, 31
Youth Group, 191

Z

Zalmay Khalilzad, 81
Zep, 27

Made in the USA
Columbia, SC
11 June 2024

36450853R00133